# Watching police,
# watching communities

# Watching police, watching communities

Mike McConville and
Dan Shepherd

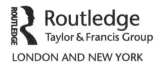

Routledge
Taylor & Francis Group

LONDON AND NEW YORK

First published 1992
by Routledge

2 Park Square, Milton Park, Abingdon, Oxon OX14 4RN
711 Third Avenue, New York, NY 10017, USA

*Routledge is an imprint of the Taylor & Francis Group,
an informa business*

First issued in paperback 2016

Transferred to Digital Printing 2005

Copyright © 1992 Mike McConville and Dan Shepherd

Typeset in Baskerville by Michael Mepham, Frome, Somerset

*British Library Cataloguing in Publication Data*
McConville, Mike
  Watching police, watching communities
  I. Title   II. Shepherd, Dan, *1962–*
  364.40458

*Library of Congress Cataloging in Publication Data*
Watching police, watching communities/Mike McConville
  and Dan Shepherd.
  p.  cm.
  Includes bibliographical references and index.
  1. Neighborhood watch programs–England–London–
  Case studies. 2. Neighborhood watch programs–Wales–
  Gwent–Case studies. 3. Neighborhood watch programs–
  England–Avon–Case studies. Neighborhood watch
  programs–England–Somerset–Case studies.
  I. Shepherd, Dan (Daniel), 1962–    . II. Title.
  HV7936.C58M38   1992
  364.4'0458'0942—dc20                                   91–29553
                                                          CIP

ISBN 978-0-415-07364-6 (hbk)
ISBN 978-1-138-98695-4 (pbk)

Every breath you take
Every move you make
Every bond you break
Every step you take

I'll be watching you

*(Sting)*

# Contents

# Contents

# Tables

# Acknowledgements

Many individuals and institutions have generously helped in this research project. The material discussed in this book arises out of a research study funded by the Barrow and Geraldine S. Cadbury Trust whose Secretary, Anthony E. Wilson, was a constant source of encouragement. We very much appreciate the understanding and support that he, and his colleague Dipali Chandra, gave us at every stage of the research. The views reported in this book are, of course, ours alone and not to be taken as the views of the trustees or staff.

The research was completely dependent upon police co-operation and we were fortunate to secure the co-operation of the Commissioner for the Police of the Metropolis, and the Chief Constables of the Avon and Somerset, and Gwent forces. The open-access policy of the police has sometimes received insufficient acknowledgement even though the mass of research studies which has produced findings highly critical of aspects of policing could well have led in other institutions to a much more defensive posture.

If force policy towards research has been praiseworthy, this has been more than matched by the reception given to researchers on the ground. In all force areas, our path was eased by designated individuals who acted as our liaison officers, helped arrange interviews, and set up beat visits. The men and women officers who constitute the core of the study went out of their way to help us, both in terms of agreeing to formal, tape-recorded, interviews and also in chatting to us informally.

In conducting the field-work and transcribing tapes, we were greatly helped by a team of friends. Ben Bowling and Mark Jackson each undertook a substantial burden of interviews with members of the public. Much of their effort involved tracking down elusive individuals and necessitated repeat visits to houses and much evening and weekend work. Both carried out the research with care and good humour. The enormous task of tape transcription and ancillary paperwork was greatly assisted by help from Jane Webb, Janet Hodgson and Angela Beuden.

We also received administrative and technical support from Ian Bryan, Caspar McConville, Sonia McConville and Satnam Singh.

Throughout the project, Aileen Stockham has acted as research secretary. We could not have wished for a more efficient, personable and intelligent secretary. Aileen has worked tirelessly on the research and she has on many occasions rescued the project in times of chaos or crisis.

We are indebted to Joe Sim for the perceptive advice and comments that he offered on the draft manuscript and to other friends and colleagues who helped us in this respect, particularly Ben Bowling, Michael Clarke and Andrew Sanders. Elisabeth Tribe at Routledge has given us strong support and helped enormously during the editorial process.

Our final thanks go to our families for supporting us over the whole period of the research.

# Chapter 1

# Crime, communities and the police

So far as the public image of British policing is concerned, the last decade has been the age of neighbourhood watch. Transplanted from the United States of America, watch schemes were introduced into Britain in the early 1980s, expanded rapidly and susbequently became the centrepiece of community crime-prevention initiatives. Neighbourhood watch was promoted as evidence of a break with a past which had been marked by fractured relations with the community, a remote police force, and styles of policing which had contributed to major confrontations with the public, including street disorders. In contrast to impositional policing, neighbourhood watch was to symbolize a new commitment to the ideals of *service*, in which the police would dedicate themselves to meeting the needs of the community at a local level. The technological age of policing in the 1960s and 1970s, in which cars, computers and radios were said to have created a metal barrier between officers and citizens, was to be replaced by a more consumer-friendly image which emphasized accessibility, approachability and partnership.

In this book we want to look at the sociological meaning behind these images. The book is not simply an examination of neighbourhood watch as a policing initiative; rather, neighbourhood watch is used as a way of looking at police–community relations and the state of contemporary policing in Britain. Thus, whilst we are concerned to look at the extent to which neighbourhood watch has penetrated into the social fabric – where schemes have taken hold and where they have failed to get off the ground; who become members and what influence schemes have upon members' attitudes and behaviour; and what, if any, impact schemes have upon crime and the fear of crime – we are also interested in the extent to which it has penetrated into policing ideologies and policing practices.

Our analysis is based upon an intensive study of neighbourhood watch and non-neighbourhood watch sites in three police forces in England and Wales over the period 1988–90. The research involved in-depth interviews with police officers, together with limited observational work, in the Metropolitan, Avon and Somerset, and Gwent police forces (see the Appendix for further research details). Within each force, research sites were chosen in consultation with the police so as to reflect the diversity of populations served and policing problems encountered, and to produce a spectrum of socio-economic, class and race dimensions.

In each of the research sites, we undertook tape-recorded interviews with samples of community beat officers (CBOs), who had amongst other duties special responsibility for neighbourhood watch schemes, and with their supervising officers and those directly responsible for co-ordinating scheme activities. In addition, we interviewed a cross-section of relief officers (ROs) whose contacts with the public are mostly confined to situations in which a member of the public calls the police for help. Whereas community beat officers are dedicated to a single beat and spend most of their time on their own, relief officers operate in groups and have a roving commission over the whole of a sub-division, including those beats of community officers. Altogether, we carried out over 200 intensive interviews with officers. We also patrolled beats with selected officers, and spent a great deal of time informally in their company.

Over the same period, we undertook a systematic survey of residents in each force, selecting areas which had neighbourhood watch schemes and comparable areas without schemes. In in-depth tape-recorded interviews, we questioned residents about their fear of crime, their knowledge and membership of neighbourhood watch, their security and surveillance practices, their relationships with the police and other related matters. As with the police, over 200 such interviews were conducted throughout the three police force areas.

Neighbourhood watch proved to be a good vantage point from which to view the questions of what the public expect of each other and of the police in a modern liberal capitalist society, as well as that of what the police expect of each other and of the public. Neighbourhood watch confronts important debates not simply about the means of policing but also about its ends; about the extent to which policing is based upon the consent of the policed; about the growth of police powers; about the degree to which policing is universally applied to all sections of society and the extent to which, if at all, there is discriminatory treatment on the basis of class, race and gender. Through neighbourhood watch, we are able to measure the temper of modern policing and to see whether there has been a significant break with the past or a continuation of traditions. Before exploring these issues in the main body of the book, however, we need to say a little about the history of neighbourhood watch in Britain.

## THE RISE OF NEIGHBOURHOOD WATCH IN BRITAIN

Neighbourhood watch (NW) was imported into Britain from the United States of America where a variety of schemes (Crime Watch, Block Watch, Community Alert, Home Watch, Neighborhood Watch and others) had been developed in the 1970s, simply as part of a much larger initiative to provide an organizational framework for citizen involvement in local crime prevention activities (Washnis, 1976; Skolnick and Bayley, 1986). The first British scheme appears to have been launched in the Cheshire village of Mollington in July 1982 (Anderton, 1985), a scheme which continues to pride itself over its 'success' in combating local crime ('Village toasts quiet victory over crime', *Guardian*, 10 August 1989). Although the South Wales Constabulary was the first British force to implement NW on a force-wide basis (Bowden, 1982), the major impetus for the spread of NW came with its adoption by the Metropolitan Police in 1983.

Inspired by the public commitment to NW of the Metropolitan Police's new Commissioner, Sir Kenneth Newman, two Metropolitan Police officers, Superintendent Turner and Detective Inspector Barker, undertook a short visit to the United States of America to study community crime prevention programmes. The resulting Turner–Barker report, based on visits to Detroit, New York, Seattle and Washington DC, recommended the establishment of pilot programmes along the lines of the Seattle model in London (Turner and Barker, 1983). Within a short time, and without the experience of pilot schemes, the Metropolitan Police launched a force-wide NW programme on 6 September 1983.

At the launch, the police stressed that, although NW would not 'solve London's crime problems' the Commissioner believed that it would 'play its part in effectively reducing the number of offences being committed – through an ever-strengthening contract between the public and the police'. (New Scotland Yard press release, 6 September 1983). Neighbourhood watch, it was stressed, was for 'ordinary home and car owners' who wanted to protect themselves and their communities from 'burglars and thieves'. Although the main emphasis was upon the prevention of burglary and the marking of property, the police felt that 'if the experience of similar schemes in America is reflected here, neighbourhood watch will make a significant impact on other types of crime, especially street robberies, thefts of and from cars and vandalism' (*ibid.*).

### The components of NW

The concept of NW is based upon the formation of a network of public-spirited members of the community who will assist the police in the fight against crime. At the launch of the Metropolitan Police scheme, emphasis was placed upon a partnership idea of policing which involved the Commissioner's model of a 'two-way notional contract between police and public'. This involved a more 'efficient and effective' use of limited resources by encouraging the public to accept a greater responsibility for preventing opportunist crime. The overall object was to make the citizen the 'eyes and ears' of the police by looking out for the unusual and reporting suspicious occurrences to the police. The principal organizational mechanism for harnessing the efforts of citizens was neighbourhood watch. According to the *Guidelines for the Introduction of Neighbourhood Watch* written by the then Chief Inspector of Constabulary, Sir Lawrence Byford, in 1985,

Neighbourhood watch is primarily a network of public spirited members of the community who observe what is going on in their own neighbourhood and report suspicious activity to the police. It involves members of the public looking out for the usual and the unusual to protect their own home and that of their neighbour, thereby reducing opportunities for criminal activity. When working effectively, neighbourhood watch can help draw the community together, making it more aware of its environment, its mutual dependence, and responsibility: in short, aiding community cohesiveness.

The official Metropolitan Police guidelines relating to NW issued in June 1983 describe the scheme as having four basic elements: first, 'neighbours watching out for each other's homes and reporting suspicious activity to the police, thereby reducing the opportunity for burglary and other crimes in the street'; secondly, 'the marking of valuable property' using a kit made freely available to the citizen; thirdly, the availability of a free home security survey carried out on request by a local crime prevention officer; and fourthly, 'the promotion of crime prevention and community campaigns to address particular local environmental issues'. Overall, therefore, the expressed aims were, by involving the public in the war against crime, to reduce crime through preventive measures and the reduction of opportunities, thereby reinforcing or creating community cohesion and lowering the fear of crime.

Individual schemes may be established either through a police initiative or as a result of citizens contacting the police. The police usually organize a launch meeting to which all residents of the target area are invited. The benefits of NW are then detailed and an attempt is made to recruit an area co-ordinator. That person will have special responsibility for liaising with the local community beat officer (CBO). Depending on the numbers of households covered, individual schemes may have a single co-ordinator or may have a substantial organization with numerous 'street co-ordinators' linking up with the area co-ordinator.

Most official pronouncements on NW, however, tend to be vague on detail and there is no clarity on what it means to have a NW scheme or to be a member of a scheme. Indeed, there is a general assumption that definition of a scheme or of membership is unnecessary either because these matters are obvious or because every scheme must be allowed to vary according to local conditions. The result is that there is no official understanding of what constitutes a scheme; what constitutes membership (whether, for example, it is personal or whether it is according to household); what responsibilities or obligations, if any, are imposed on citizens by membership; and what responsibilities or obligations, if any, are imposed on the police by the creation of an official scheme. Thus, it is unclear what is meant when it is claimed that over three and a half million households are covered by NW (*Guardian*,

10 August 1989). And what does a person have to do in order to qualify as a member: Attend an inaugural meeting? Attend meetings regularly? Be on a co-ordinator's membership list? Place stickers in a window? Undertake surveillance activity? Live in a road where there is a scheme?

Answers to these kinds of question are important in thinking about NW. There is, for example, little purpose in collecting official figures on the number of schemes if there is no agreement about or understanding of what exactly is being counted (cf. Husain and Bright, 1990). Moreover, any analysis which seeks to measure the crime prevention impact of NW must be flawed if it does not take into account the differences between schemes. And any measurement of crime prevention must tease out what, if anything, acts as a deterrent to would-be criminals – stickers, signs, surveillance activity of residents, patrolling, increased security systems. On issues of this sort, official accounts of NW are unhelpful.

### 'Success' and the growth of schemes

Within a very short time of its launch, NW was officially portrayed as a success. Assistant Commissioner Wilford Gibson was reported to have claimed a 'dramatic' reduction in burglaries in the Hurlingham area of Fulham, London, as a result of NW (*Standard*, 31 May 1984), and Metropolitan officers estimated reductions of crime of between 10 and 60 per cent (*Standard*, 5 November 1984). According to Superintendent Brian Turner, one of the authors of the influential Turner–Barker report of 1983, the benefits of NW included: 'more information about what's going on in the community and the information is of better quality. So we are able to defeat the criminal by securing convictions much more easily' (London Weekend Television, *The London Programme*, 4 January 1985).

The story of success is strongly reflected in individual NW newsletters, most of which are published by or in conjunction with the local police, as the following examples illustrate:

Neighbourhood watch is here to stay and for us it has worked with a tremendous drop in the burglary rate and many success stories.

(South Norwood, London, *Neighbourhood Watch Newsletter*, 1988 issue)

We have already achieved a marked decrease in crime and an excellent detection rate with our neighbourhood watch. . . . Burglary is down again for the second year running and we are sure that neighbourhood watch played its part in obtaining this further reduction.

(West Midlands Police, *Watchwords*, March 1989)

'Neighbourhood Watch Schemes definitely help to reduce crime in their areas, especially burglaries' says Detective Inspector Tom McNally. 'To begin with Neighbourhood Watch Schemes became very much more security conscious and fitted good locks and bolts to their doors and windows. This deterred the thief, and there was about a 25 per cent reduction in burglaries on our police area between 1986 and 1987. Now the Neighbourhood Watch Schemes are helping to solve burglaries as well, with the detection rate for the first five months of 1988 twice that for the same period in 1987'.

(Avon and Somerset Constabulary, *Neighbourhood Watch News*: 4)

A similar picture is put forward by government ministers. After a somewhat cautious start, ministers have become increasingly bullish in their support for NW and have advanced strong claims for its success. Thus, one year after the Metropolitan Police launch of NW, Giles Shaw MP, then Minister of State at the Home Office was cautiously optimistic: 'Whilst it is too early to draw firm general conclusions, initial indications are that neighbourhood watch schemes have reduced crime and increased detection of offenders by the police' (Home Office, *News Release*, 19 October 1984). Five years later the then Minister of State at the Home Office, John Patten MP, was much more enthusiastic about what, he said, had become 'an unstoppable movement':

It must be more than a coincidence that our most recent crime figures showed a substantial decrease in property crime. We have always known that community crime prevention is a force for the good – bringing neighbours together, leading to good relations with the police and reducing fear of crime and we hoped that it would help to reduce crime itself. Our own statistics, coupled with the enthusiastic support of the public, now seem to be proving this to be the case.

(Home Office, *News Release*, 8 August 1989)

Media coverage has substantially reinforced this picture, although some concerns and reservations have been voiced. The association of NW with the property-owning classes was acknowledged by the police to be a drawback at an early stage: 'The middle-class image', said Superintendent Turner, 'is a problem – it had that image in the States' (*Guardian*, 4 July 1984). This led to the belief of 'many officers' that NW 'will be much more difficult to set up in the areas where they are most needed such as the vast down-at-heel council estates' (*The Times*, 10 February 1984). Subsequently, concerns surfaced over the preventive role of NW and over 'political' obstacles to its spread. Thus, in 1986 it was reported that 'neighbourhood watches to deter criminals are to be given a shake-up by Scotland Yard after evidence that they are transferring crime elsewhere and turning burglars into muggers' (*The Sunday Times*, 1 June 1986). And throughout there has been an undercurrent of concern at the political nature of NW. An editorial in *The Times* bluntly put one point of view shortly after the launch of NW by the Metropolitan Police:

> There exists a small body of left-wingers who will treat the scheme not as the beginnings of the busybody state, but the police state. Their animus against the police is such that, as socialists allegedly devoted to the well-being of the common people, they have allowed their priorities to be distorted. They show, for example, scant concern for the elderly who are virtually house-bound not through infirmity but because they live on crime-afflicted estates. If the effectiveness of urban policing is diminished, for them there is no hope in their declining years. For them, a watch scheme is a potential godsend.
>
> (*The Times*, 8 September 1983)

This has been followed up by complaints from the police (*The Sunday Times*, 16 October 1988) and from government ministers (*Guardian*, 12 July 1989) that some Labour-controlled local authorities are obstructing the spread of NW.

But concerns of these kinds have been subordinated to a general claim of success. Given the background story of 'success' in deterring criminals, boosting detection rates, and bringing neighbours together, it is hardly surprising that NW appears to have grown rapidly from modest beginnings, as Table 1.1 demonstrates.

*Table 1.1* The growth of neighbourhood watch schemes according to official figures

| Date | Number of schemes |
| --- | --- |
| 1985 (July) | 1,300 |
| 1987 (March) | 18,000 |
| 1989 (July) | 66,000 |
| 1990 (March) | 81,302 |
| 1991 (March) | 91,000 |

Source: *New Society*, 20.9.1985; *The Times*, 6.3.1987, *Guardian*, 12.7.1989; *Guardian*, 2.3.1990; *Daily Mail*, 10.4.1991

Proponents of NW who are close to official thinking have predicted that there will be perhaps 120,000 schemes by the mid-1990s (Bright and Husain, 1990). Even without the benefit of research evidence, however, there are several reasons why these official figures and what they might signify should be treated with caution. In the first place, whilst the figures depict a story of continuous success, it is obvious that some schemes never really get off the ground and that others, even if successfully launched, soon become dormant. This is not, of course, a particular criticism of NW but merely a statement of what we know of all such informal social organizations. In the second place, the basis of the official figures has been challenged as exaggerating the numbers of new schemes ('Home Office inflated watchdog figures', *The Observer*, 27 August 1989). Thus, for example, an increase of 100 new schemes in Avon and Somerset was reported by the Home Office as an increase of 772, and whilst the Home Office claimed that there were 227 new schemes in the Metropolitan Police District over the period March–June 1989, the Metropolitan Police said that statistics of this kind had not been collated.

The official statistics need also to be treated with caution because they imply that NW has a universal appeal and that its spread across the country is unrelated to socio-economic and sociopolitical factors. The emphasis upon home security and property ownership would suggest, however, that NW would be more likely to take hold in some areas (such as home-owning, economically advantaged and stable communities) and less likely to succeed in others (characterized, for example, by rented accommodation, economically disadvantaged individuals and shifting populations). Moreover, insofar as NW has been initiated and promoted by the police, it cannot be taken for granted that the police would make equivalent (or greater) efforts to establish NW in areas (such as some traditional working-class communities) where their own legitimacy is contested and where their presence is accepted only reluctantly.

## THE IMPACT OF NW

As represented in official statements, NW is not meant to be simply another bureaucratic organization grafted on to the existing police delivery system. Instead, it locks into claims about a new kind of policing model which moves the emphasis away from the imposition of social control and the crude measurement of success by arrest rates, and towards a service model which puts the needs of the community at the top of the policing agenda and gives recognition to the benefits of good police–community relations. Apart from influencing the behaviour of potential criminals, NW is, therefore, intended to have a direct impact upon both the community and the police.

### The community

The conceptual thinking behind NW is that the creation of a scheme will, or is very likely to, effect a number of beneficial changes in the behaviour of residents. These changes include: improving household security; increasing personal safety measures; and heightening an individual's social awareness and civic responsibility, by setting up positive relationships with neighbours and by engaging in watching or surveillance activities.

It is not clear from official pronouncements, however, how a person's behaviour should in fact change. One message, for example, encourages a greater awareness of possible threats or danger, which would be expected to lead to more cautious behaviour, producing, in extreme cases, a 'fortress mentality'. On the other hand, part of the message of NW is to reduce the fear of crime by educating people about the 'real', rather than imagined, risks of victimization in their locality; this message might encourage people in some areas to take fewer precautionary measures as a result of a more 'realistic' assessment of risk.

A second set of claims relating to the community is concerned with changes in the relationship of residents with the police. The 'social contract' claim is that NW is a partnership in which the community and the police share, or come to share, a mutual concern about crime. Insofar as police–community relations are deficient, NW is intended to repair and confirm the positive aspects. In this perspective, community policing is intended to transform policing *of* the community into policing *for* the community.

This second set of claims is also problematic. In the first place, it tends to view the community as homogenous, whereas we know that many communities are beset with conflicting interests. Secondly, whilst eschewing an impositional style of policing, it rests the partnership model upon a common concern over crime. The belief that crime is a major concern of the community is, however, an assumption rather than an established fact. This latter point is important because programmes could easily fail if citizens are not centrally concerned about crime.

**The police**

Embedded in official representations about NW are claims about the police which are part of a response to the crisis of legitimacy faced by the police in the 1970s and early 1980s. That crisis centred upon a system of policing which was increasingly seen to be: coercive in nature – most clearly dramatized in the accelerating deployment of riot-trained specialist squads such as the Special Patrol Group; lacking accountability – with the autonomy of chief constables a matter of concern, and a complaints system which lacked the confidence of both the public and police officers themselves; badly underperforming in terms of preventing and clearing crime – with official statistics recording an inexorable rise in reported crime and a declining clear-up rate by the police; and losing the public's confidence – with a particularly dramatic decline in relations with the black community, itself a factor in the street riots of 1981 (for perspectives on these issues see Campbell,

1980; Bridges and Bunyan, 1983; Gordon, 1984; Reiner, 1985). Whilst the police have sought to address these issues in a variety of other ways, NW encapsulates the thrust of the police approach and epitomizes the promise of a new age of policing.

This new age is to be marked, in the first place, by an emphasis upon *consensual* policing. NW rhetoric is underpinned by a commitment to talk to the community with a view to identifying community concerns so that these can be appropriately addressed. This is reinforced by the commitment to shift resources towards community-based officers whose morale and status are also to be raised. There is also much talk of a contract with the public, and of a partnership in constructing a consensual policing model. A remote and distant body is to change into 'the listening force'. This, in turn, implies a system of local accountability, designed as part of the answer to criticisms that the police had become an autonomous body in society, able to create and implement crucial changes in policy without going through the political process.

In response to the allegations that the police were really only interested in social control and the management of public order, the new policing espoused not only an interest in crime but also a concern about crime. The police were now prepared to concede that they alone could not contain crime but they promised that, with the help of the community, they would do something about crime by taking it seriously. This new model was to be available to all, irrespective of class, race and gender, and past problems with black communities in particular would be repaired by ridding their neighbourhoods of crime and establishing a system of *sensitive* policing.

### Coercive and sensitive policing in parallel

Of course, even at a conceptual rather than an empirical level, claims of this sort are highly problematic. The new community policing was never promised as a replacement for other more coercive styles but as complementary, and special para-military support units might be renamed but would otherwise continue. Whilst official pronouncements stressed 'crime concern', there was no promise of an institutional shift away from the historical emphasis upon clear-up rates towards crime prevention. Moreover, there was every reason to suppose that unanchored commitments to increase the status of beat officers within the police would struggle for success, in the way that similar commitments had in the past. And without an institutional commitment to root out racism within the ranks of the police, the prospects for a sea-change in police relations with ethnic minorities were not good.

### Fear and crime

In addition, central to NW and to many of the other community policing initiatives is an untested belief about fear of crime. The whole edifice of NW rests on the assumption that fear of crime is so prevalent that citizens can be easily mobilized by a rhetoric which promises action against crime. This assumption was especially easy for the police to make because they had for a very long time sought to locate their own legitimacy not in their public order and social control functions but instead in their efficiency in waging the war against crime (Manning, 1977). The soundness of the police assumption about public concern over routine crime is, however, called into question by the fact that they have often felt it necessary to obtain public sanction to extend their powers by creating a 'moral panic' over specific issues, such as in the 'mugging' scare of the 1970s (Hall et al., 1978). The central importance accorded to crime in this new policing system is, therefore, problematic.

These and related issues emerge as underlying themes throughout the rest of this book. The partnership basis of NW raises the question of public expectations of the police, a matter addressed in Chapter 2. In Chapter 3, we deal with fear of crime, the issue upon which mobilization of the public essentially depends. Chapter 4 examines how NW is working in practice, the extent to which citizens are 'active' and engage in surveillance and other activities; and it looks at sites where NW has not taken hold to see if they differ in any important ways from NW sites. In Chapter 5 we look at how the different police forces have addressed the challenge of NW and examine, within individual forces, the kinds of officer undertaking beat work, the emphasis they give to NW, and the success they have in establishing and servicing schemes. Some of the themes which emerge in the review of the police response are pursued in Chapters 6 and 7, which deal with the obstacles to community policing within police culture and discuss why, despite the hierarchical structure of the police, official pronouncements of reform fail to influence the attitudes and behaviour of the lower ranks. Finally, in Chapter 8, we draw together some of the findings and look at what the NW programme tells us about the structure of the police force and the nature of policing in contemporary Britain.

# Chapter 2

# Public satisfaction and dissatisfaction with the police

Public attitudes towards the police are fundamental towards successful policing. This is clearly acknowledged in the official conceptualization of NW as involving and promoting a 'partnership' approach to crime prevention, and in the recognition that public trust and confidence in the police must be maintained and deepened. The police are heavily dependent upon the public to provide information about criminal incidents and upon their willingness to act as witnesses in court proceedings, both matters predicated upon positive police–public relations. Public evaluations and expectations of the police are thus critical to understanding the likely success of specific policing initiatives like NW and of policing efforts in general.

In this chapter, we explore public attitudes to the local police. Our analysis arises out of our survey of residents in which we asked respondents: Are you satisfied with your local police? Taking everything into account, would you say that the police in this area do a good job or a bad job? Are there any changes you would like to see in policing this area? The level of public satisfaction with the existing service is clearly an important factor in debates about planned or possible changes to policing, and is worth exploring in detail. In follow-up questions we explored public attitudes to foot patrols, since this issue is intimately connected with the conception of home beats and other kinds of locally-based officer. We are less concerned with overall levels of satisfaction with the police or with levels of support for car or foot patrols than with what lies behind public satisfaction or dissatisfaction with the police, and why people might value a particular form of patrol. Thus, whilst research has, as we shall see, demonstrated a clear public demand for foot patrols, there has been no systematic information, as Weatheritt (1987) points out, on what accounts for this demand.

Before examining the results of our survey in detail, there are some important points that need to be borne in mind in interpreting public attitudes towards the police. The most fundamental point is the importance of avoiding simple answers and absolutist conceptions. Policing is, as Reiner (1985, p. 50) points out, 'an inherently conflict-ridden enterprise'. This arises not simply out of the fact that an officer, no matter how benign, always possesses a monopoly on the potential use of legitimate force (Bittner, 1967; Punch, 1979), but also from the variety of functions an officer may perform, from the contradictory expectations that may be held about the purposes of policing, and from the different ways in which police–public encounters may be generated.

It would be unrealistic, therefore, to expect either universal approval of the police or unqualified support for all aspects of policing witnessed, imagined or experienced. The nature of a motoring encounter with the police (which accounts for a large proportion of public-police contacts) can, for example, confirm or dispel a previously-held attitude about police behaviour or style *in general*, not simply in relation to motoring matters. Moreover, some residents might misjudge police action or interpret it in the light of biases they hold for or against the police. Whilst the in-depth interview helps to detect the more obvious biases, these limitations remain in all perceptual research.

A second point to notice is the difference between public attitudes to law and order, and criticisms that might be entertained of the police. It would be a serious misunderstanding to equate people's identification of shortcomings in the police with some unexplicated rejection of the values of law, order and the value of a policed society. Even radical critics of the police generally seek change *in* the police rather than abolition *of* the police.

## PUBLIC SATISFACTION WITH THE POLICE

Over the last thirty years, surveys have consistently shown a very broad degree of public satisfaction with the police. Thus, the Royal Commission on the Police (1962) conducted a national opinion survey which resulted in what the Commission described as 'an overwhelming vote of confidence in the police'. Detailed figures showed that some 85 per cent of the professional and managerial classes, and some 82 per cent of the skilled, semi-skilled and unskilled working classes had 'great respect' for the police. Results obtained in a later survey by Shaw and Williamson (1972) were broadly similar (see Reiner, 1985, p. 50; and cf. Brogden, 1982, p.204). More recently, however, studies have uncovered marked differences between groups, with substantial evidence of significant levels of dissatisfaction in urban areas, and a decline in the general level of satisfaction with the police.

Discussing the results of the first British Crime Survey, Hough and Mayhew (1983) report that for public-initiated contacts, about 80 per cent of those who approached the police other than as victims found the police to be helpful and pleasant. There were, however, marked differences between groups: older people were more satisfied than younger, women more than men, and non-manual workers more than manual. Police in rural areas were rated higher than those in more urban areas. Of police-initiated contacts, 8 per cent of women over 60 said that they had received some impolite treatment from the police, a figure that rose to 52 per cent among young men (ibid., p. 30). This broad pattern was supported in the surveys conducted by Bennett (1990) in Acton and Wimbledon. Bennett found that older respondents rated the police more highly than younger, female more highly than male, and white more highly than non-white (ibid., pp. 121–2).

Research undertaken in urban areas has disclosed serious levels of dissatisfaction among some sections of the community. The Policy Studies Institute (1983), for example, found a 'dangerous lack of confidence' in the police among substantial numbers of young white people and a 'disastrous lack of confidence' among young people of West Indian origin. But the study also found that this did not amount to a rejection of the present system of policing: Afro-Caribbeans were just as likely as whites to report victimization to the police, and were willing (at least to some extent) to co-operate with the police (ibid., vol. IV, pp. 332–3). Similarly, both Islington Crime Surveys (Jones et al., 1986; Crawford et al., 1990) found considerable dissatisfaction with regard to local policing, that it is concentrated most heavily in young people, and that it is growing (Crawford et al., 1990, p. 103). The later survey showed that crime was a central concern of the people of Islington, and that a substantial (and increasing) majority of people saw the police as unsuccessful in dealing with crime (ibid., Tables 2.8 and 4.17).

The broadest measurement over time of support for the police is found in the three British Crime Surveys carried out in 1982, 1984 and 1988. In the first, 92 per cent of the residents of England and Wales who had an opinion about the police rated their performance as good or very good, a figure that dropped to 90 per cent in 1984, and to 85 per cent in 1988. Moreover, the percentage giving the police the highest marks has dropped from 43 per cent in 1982 to only 25 per cent in 1988. Summarizing the findings, Skogan (1990) states that the surveys

> indicate that confidence has fallen in almost every type of community and in many important social categories. The percentage of persons who think police do a 'very good job' has declined the most in small towns and rural areas, among women and the elderly, and among whites – all groups which traditionally have been the most supportive of the police.
>
> (ibid., p. 2)

This decline in public satisfaction with the police is consistent with the findings of opinion polls conducted by independent organizations. Thus, MORI reported a decline in public satisfaction from 75 per cent to 58 per cent between 1981 and 1989 (MORI, 1989). This decline in public confidence leading to calls for a royal commission into policing (*Guardian*, editorial, 2 April 1991), has been recognized by the police themselves. For example, the Chief Constable of Derbyshire, reflecting on almost thirty years' experience, stated that the fall in public confidence in the police 'is more severe than any I can remember' (*Guardian*, 28 November 1990).

Whilst our own research fits in at various points with earlier studies, we wish to re-emphasize the problems of measurement. The contradictory nature of policing makes it difficult for people to provide the dichotomized responses so favoured by social scientists. Thus people were able to say, quite properly, that they were satisfied with the police and then go on to make scathing criticisms of the attitudes or behaviour of police officers. Responses of an opposite kind were also encountered. The position adopted here by respondents is a result partly of the psychological difficulty of being objective about an institution that is supposed to be viewed in a favourable light, and partly of the problems in assessing an institution with multiple and often contradictory functions. It follows therefore that general findings which are set out in Table 2.1 need to be understood in terms of the ensuing discussion rather than given an importance in their own right.

*Table 2.1*  Overall levels of satisfaction with local police by force area

| Force area | Satisfied % | Dissatisfied % | Ambivalent % | Don't know % |
|---|---|---|---|---|
| Gwent | 58.7 | 21.7 | 6.5 | 13.1 |
| Avon and | | | | |
| Somerset | 34.6 | 30.8 | 19.2 | 15.4 |
| Metropolitan | 31.6 | 28.2 | 22.2 | 18.0 |

*Note*: 'Ambivalent' refers to those who offered both praise and criticism of the police, but who did not say if they were satisfied or dissatisfied.

As Table 2.1 discloses, satisfaction with the local police was highest in Gwent, with broadly similar levels found for both Avon and Somerset and the Metropolitan police. Substantial differences emerged between areas within each force. Rural and suburban areas tended to have higher levels of satisfaction than inner-city areas, but there were in all areas occasionally substantial differences between roads that in other respects appeared identical. There were also marked differences in response according to demographic characteristics. Of those who expressed themselves to be satisfied or dissatisfied with their local police, higher levels of satisfaction were reported by whites (59.6 per cent) as against black people (46.7 per cent), old (67.9 per cent) as against young (40.0 per cent), and female (68.1 per cent) as against male (57.4 per cent). These findings are consistent with the results of the third British Crime Survey which found 'a large gulf between whites and racial minorities, and between younger and older people, in their degree of satisfaction with police contacts' (Skogan, 1990, p. 13 and Table 4). We discuss below what lies behind some of these broad expressions of satisfaction or dissatisfaction.

**Non-committal**

A handful of people in each police force area felt unable to decide whether or not they were satisfied with the police. This was not based upon indifference towards the police, but rather arose from lack of substantial contacts with the police. Although a significant minority of adults approach the police on some matters each year, such as requesting directions, reporting missing property or asking for help (40 per cent in the first British Crime Survey: Hough and Mayhew, 1983), and about one in five are approached by the police, a lot of people still have no contact at all with the police or ones of a fleeting and inconsequential nature. The following quotations illustrate responses of residents in this category:

*Gwent rural resident*
We've had nothing to do with the local police, so it's very difficult to say whether we are satisfied or not. Inadequate experience!

*Avon and Somerset suburban resident*
I don't know. There isn't a local police station in [the area], so I don't think the people [here] see that there are police here. They don't seem to actually exist, they're not noticeable in the job that they are doing.

*Metropolitan suburban resident*
I've never seen them. You see the odd squad car drive round the [nearby] estate. . . . I just don't know enough about the police in this area to say whether I'm satisfied.

**Positive evaluations: no experience**

Even though they had enjoyed little or no contact with the police, a larger group of people none the less regarded their local police with satisfaction. Two principal strands of reasoning underlay these evaluations. First, residents were prepared to express themselves as satisfied because, in the absence of contacts, they had no reason to be dissatisfied. Second, psychologically predisposed to support the police, many were able to hold on to an idealized representation of policing precisely because it was unanchored in, and uncontroverted by, experience. By comparison, we found few people in this category who held a negative view of the police. These results are consistent with the findings of the third British Crime Survey that those who did not have personal experience of the police but relied upon television, radio and newspapers as their sources of information, were more positive in their assessment of police performance (Skogan, 1990, p. 19). The exceptions here, which we deal with in a later section in this chapter, are residents who complain of the lack of contact with the police.

*Metropolitan suburban resident*
Q: Are you satisfied with your local police?

A: Yes, definitely.

Q: Why do you say that?

A: Really you know, we don't have much call to be in contact with the police. Fortunately, touch wood, we've never had any reason to rely on the police in any way. But I am sure from what I know of the police that they would be totally reliable.

Q: What sort of policing would you like to see in this area?

A: To be honest, I really don't know what kind of policing we've got here. I never see a police officer in this area. Come to think of it, I don't think I ever see one.

*Gwent rural resident*

Yes, satisfied, but again it is a bit of a non-event. Satisfied, more by omission than by commission, because I've had no call to use them. I've no complaints about them.

Although they had had no personal experience of policing, these residents appealed to an image of policing which they believed to be current today or strongly empathized with the job of the police ('Bearing in mind the job they have to do nowadays' and 'I think they have a difficult job' were typical expressions).

## Positive experiences of the police

The residue who expressed satisfaction with the local police were people who had had some form of contact with the police and had considered this to be valuable. There were two distinct groups involved here. The first were those people who had come into contact with the police as victims of crime. The second were those who knew local officers or who saw them frequently. So far as victims are concerned, our findings are broadly consistent with those of earlier studies which found that a large proportion of police–victim contacts are positive. Thus, Hough and Mayhew (1983), reporting on the first British Crime Survey data, found that four-fifths of those victims who had any contact with the police over their case expressed satisfaction. Data from the third British Crime Survey do show, however, a significant fall-off in levels of victim satisfaction (Mayhew *et al.*, 1989). Work on victims of violent offences by Shapland (1982) and on burglary victims by Maguire (1982) found that the primary causes of dissatisfaction were an unsympathetic manner and a failure to keep victims informed.

Although, as we shall see, people do not have high expectations of what the police can do in solving crimes, many of those who reported some form of prior victimization said that they were happy with the service given by the police. Responses of the following kinds were encountered in all police force areas:

> When I was burgled the police were really helpful. They sent the crime prevention guy round and he then advised on things to put on doors at the back and at the front. They were very helpful.

> I'm satisfied with them. I've only dealt with them once when I had a bicycle stolen from the railway station and they were quite efficient.

> They have been pretty good to us after [the burglary], and they have come out to other people I know who have had problems. A friend who lived in [another road], they sent the Victim Support group round, and stuff like this. They seemed to be aware of what they can offer people.

The other significant group were those who were satisfied with their local police precisely because they saw them as *local* police. There can be no doubt whatsoever, as we shall see later in this chapter, that there is a very strong public demand for local policing. People want to identify with the police, to be able to approach the police easily and without apprehension, and to know who their local police are. Although there were isolated examples of people remarking on the local nature of the policing in the other two forces, this positive response was a characteristic of the sub-urban and rural sites of Gwent. In these areas, the police were considered by residents to be *their* police. This was, of course, assisted by the fact that some of the sites were served by one officer, but there was a general feeling (except in the inner-city Gwent area) that Gwent police were accessible and were concerned for the community. The following quotations from Gwent residents illustrate this very positive sentiment towards the police:

> Our local police constable does a good job.

> I am satisfied with the local police. He's a very pleasant police-man. I'm quite happy with what we've got and the kids respect him.

Gwent police are tremendous.

This constable we've got, he's excellent. It's not only me; he goes round and speaks to you. If you've got any complaint, you go to him, he'll see to it and come back to you and tell you what he'd done. He's absolutely bloody marvellous.

Testimonies of this sort point up a theme that is of fundamental importance in the public's evaluation of policing and in the changes they would like brought about in policing methods and styles: there is a widespread and persistent demand for policing of a local and personal character.

### Dissatisfaction with the police

A very substantial degree of dissatisfaction with the police was evident from our interviews with residents, especially but not exclusively in the Metropolitan and Avon and Somerset Forces. Three broad strands of criticism were discernible: the lack of visibility of the police; the lack of interpersonal skills of individual officers; and the failure of the police to keep in step with community needs and wishes.

Many people complained about not seeing the police or seeing them in settings which made personal contact impossible. Although, as we have seen, people in rural areas tended to give very positive evaluations of the police because they identified with individual officers, there was still a sense in some rural people of remoteness from the police. This arose principally because they did not have an officer *resident* in the village or because the nearest station was considered to be too far away from the community it served. These feelings were echoed in suburban areas which had lost local stations as a result of 'rationalization' of police services. Overall, this group was characterized by a demand for local police who could be seen to belong to the area policed:

*Gwent rural resident*
I am not satisfied for the simple reason that to get our local police we have to 'phone four miles. There's no local policeman as such. We have a policeman's house on the [nearby] main road, but he's not for us.

*Avon and Somerset suburban resident*
We never see them! There's no local nick. You couldn't run up

there if you needed them. I have never looked out of the window and seen a policeman walking up and down the road.

*London suburban resident*
I am not satisfied with the police. I think they do a bad job because I don't see any round here.

This perception of the public was most strikingly displayed in public-sector housing areas, most noticeable in the inner-city council estate area of Gwent. Here the police were generally rated as doing a 'bad job' precisely because they were said to under-police the area. Residents felt that the police were not interested in and did not care about the problems of the estate. The police sub-station, which was not staffed for much of the time, symbolized for residents the lack of interest by the police in the estate:

If I saw them I'd say they do a good job, but I don't see them.

We have a police station down there, and if you look down there, it's locked up. What good is it? All they do is waste people's money.

It's diabolical. There's police offices over there and none of them are used.

Every time I want to go in the police station it's never open. I was going to go in and find out about [the research] but it's very rare they are in.

They do a bad job. . . . They don't bother as such; they are not really interested.

Another group of residents were critical of the police on the basis of a perceived lack of interpersonal skills. This finding echoes the third British Crime Survey's finding (Mayhew *et al.*, 1989) of a consistent drop in satisfaction across all types of victimization. Mayhew *et al.* (1989) report the main reasons why respondents said they were dissatisfied as being that the police did not do enough, showed a lack of interest, and failed to keep the respondent informed (Table A.9, Appendix A). The inability of some officers to chat to members of the public, take a sympathetic line on distressing matters, and to radiate confidence in the way they handle incidents, was often remarked upon by senior officers to whom we spoke and was echoed in the views of residents. Encounters with the public are infrequent and short-lived when they

do take place. The manner and attitude of an officer can, therefore, quickly generate a favourable or unfavourable image of
police in general. In addition to this, some residents said that
officers were in general deficient in communication skills or were
not interested in establishing relations with members of the public.
Some of these points are illustrated in the following quotations:

> Generally you couldn't stop and talk to them just off the cuff or
> strike up a conversation about something. If there's something
> going on and you ask them 'what's going on?' they just don't
> seem to want to bother explaining to the general public.

> The ones I've met are quite frankly educationally subnormal.
> They seem rather stupid to me. . . . I mean, [at the NW meet-
> ing] we were all sniggering and giggling because they could
> barely string two words together.

Some officers were described as 'rude', younger officers sometimes
gave the impression of being 'flash' or 'Jack the lads in uniform',
and others were thought of as 'unsympathetic' or 'bullies'.

A third source of general dissatisfaction with the police, eman-
ating from all sections of the community, came from a feeling that
the police did not reflect the needs and wishes of the community.
These criticisms took a variety of forms: a concern in the Metropolitan and Avon and Somerset areas that the police force failed
to reflect the multiracial character of the community; a concern in
all areas that the police spent too much time on certain matters
such as motoring offences; and a concern, in Avon and Somerset
and the Metropolitan Police district, about police accountability.
Later in the chapter we shall deal in more detail with serious
complaints in London and Avon and Somerset about policing
styles, but we can note here that the policing of public order
situations and the practice of stop-searches attracted widespread
condemnation. We give below a selection of views of residents from
all three force areas on some of these matters:

> The police just don't understand what people think and feel.
> Do you see any policeman knocking on doors and asking what
> we would like and the service that we pay for with our taxes?
> Accountability!

> They should spend a bit more time on protecting homes and
> cars rather than going after the motorists who may be speeding.

It's a multi-racial area and I haven't seen any black police since I came [here]. I think any sort of police force if it's patrolling a suburban area has to be almost a part of the community, otherwise it won't be accepted. From what I know of [this area] that's half the problem.

Obviously most people would say they would want to see more police on the beat and stuff like that, and I would accept that. But with the police attitude at the moment, with them walking up and down the street I would feel more threatened by them than comforted by them really. The amount of times I have been stopped and searched while I have been out and all sorts of things. Anything from minor things to being arrested and actually being locked up for a few hours and things like that. It doesn't make me feel more comfortable having people wandering the streets doing that. I would actually like someone wandering the streets making me feel more secure but in the current sort of set-up it's just not going to happen with the attitudes they have got.

### How the public rate the police: ideals and reality

In this section we begin to explore the basis upon which residents evaluate their police. An understanding of the basis of residents' evaluation helps in deciding what weight should be given to their views and what kind of response they should generate. If, for example, residents have wholly unrealistic expectations as to what kind of service their local police can deliver, criticisms of the police for failing to live up to these expectations should be given less weight than those which are better grounded. Here we explore the extent to which residents' evaluations are based upon some unrealizable standard, and the extent to which there is an appreciation of limitations on what the police are able to achieve.

Perhaps surprisingly, we found little evidence of an appeal to a 'golden past' among residents of any age grouping underlying their judgement of the local police. Occasionally, residents would refer to how 'policing used to be' or what it was like 'years ago' and in a couple of interviews 'Dixon of Dock Green' made an appearance. However, these images were almost never used to judge the police of today, principally because those who invoked the images of the past regarded previous times as irrevocably lost; 'those days will never come back', 'it'll never be like that again' typified the thinking of residents. Where they were evoked, visions of the past were used to reinforce a demand for officers who were locally-based and who would be known in the community:

*Gwent resident*
Q: Are you satisfied with the local police?
A: Yes, I don't know any policemen who live in the area or anything like that. Obviously some do, I suppose, but you don't recognise them now like you used to do years ago. Years ago you knew them and would speak to them; they seldom speak now.
Q: How long ago was this?
A: Before and after the war. They used to walk around, you see: Constable so and so, and Sergeant so and so. They'd come in and have a chat. This changed I suppose in the middle 50s. Gradually the police disappeared off the roads, cars came in and you lost the constable on the street. Kids would play 'kick the tin' in the road and he'd come and you'd run like hell. Now, you wouldn't see one now.

*London resident*
It would be nice if the police could get down into the street. It would be nice to have a cop wandering up and down here occasionally, if we all knew his name it would be nice. And if we thought a cop lived quite close, *if one did*!, it might be useful to know where he lived or something. He should get to know the kids and be a friend rather than someone who is always looking for trouble. When I was a girl, a policeman was someone who was always going to help you out; now, he is someone who is going to nab you.

*Avon and Somerset resident*
I don't know if it is possible but I'd like to see maybe working back to the traditional sort of policing where the policemen were people from the community who knew you.

The nature of residents' concerns also derives from their 'under-standing' of police resources and the police capacity to solve crime. Many residents reasoned that their expectations of the police had to be seen against the resources which were available to the police. The police, like the other institutions of law and order such as the prisons, have assiduously pushed the line that they lack resources even though there has been a vast increase, in both staffing and financial terms, during the 1980s. In all force areas, residents' judgements about the quality of the service presently delivered, and demands for improved service were mediated by the belief that the police were hampered by shortages of personnel, equipment and finance. Opinion surveys which uncover complaints that the police did not arrive fast enough (for example, the third British Crime Survey found this true of 14 per cent of those who had a specific complaint about police service: Skogan, 1990) have to be read against a broader public perception of the demands on the police. Complaints about response times are often complaints about police resources, rather than the police service.

> Q: Are you satisfied with your local police?
> A: Well I am, I guess, but they are over-extended in this part of the world.
> Q: What do you mean?
> A: Well, for example, I had someone attempt to break into my house earlier this year. Fortunately, they weren't successful. I contacted the police, they took four hours to attend and then I was supposed to have back-up visits a couple of days later which didn't materialize. And obviously they'd got more important things to do, which I accept.

> I think they do as much as their resources allow them to do. I mean, I don't know whether they are short-staffed or what; I should imagine they probably are. I'm sure they do a pretty good job under somewhat extreme circumstances.

> The service doesn't seem good but that is most probably because they are understaffed.

A similar picture emerged in relation to the police capacity to solve crime. In general, people do not hold exaggerated views as to the detection ability of the police in relation to standard burglaries, thefts and similar offences. Research into the non-reporting of 'crimes', for example, shows that a significant feature in the victim's decision not to report a crime is a feeling that the police would not have been able to do anything about the incident (Skogan, 1984; Mayhew et al., 1989), and we found that this was also true of many of those who had made a report to the police. Of course, this is in part a result of what residents are told by the police who, it seems, are careful to explain to people at the scene of many kinds of incident, such as burglary, thefts, and criminal damage, that there is no likelihood of discovering the culprit. Even where residents expressed concern at police efficiency in this respect, this was almost invariably moderated by an appreciation of the difficulties confronting the police:

> I think, certainly from my neighbours who've been burgled on a number of occasions now, I don't think they're particularly satisfied with the criminal detection ability of the police. But then that's an enormously difficult job because there are thousands of burglaries going on every day of the week.

> I'm satisfied [with the police] to the extent that when we had the burglary they were round, they took fingerprints. I knew they weren't going to get anywhere but they did all the right things.

> I think it's become clear to the general public that the police really don't have a dramatic effect on crime, because when you get down to a minor crime, like burglary, then there are so many of them and there are so many possible culprits in urban areas such as this, there is no way any one particular crime will be traced back. The clear-up rate for a particular crime is going to be minimal. So that seems to have become more obvious to people.

What was true of detection was also true of deterrence. While there was an occasional expression of the view that the police could, by increasing their visibility, deter crime, most people felt that there was little that the police could do to reduce the crime rate. 'I don't honestly think you're going to deter people who've got intentions of committing a crime like burglary' and 'To expect the police to maintain sufficient presence to actually prevent burglary is impossible', were typical comments of residents.

Contrary to the assertions of senior police officers that public expectations of what the police can do are unrealistic (a speaker at the ACPO conference quoted in the *Guardian*, 18 June 1987), it is clear, therefore, that public conceptions of the police show an appreciation of the realities of modern society and are not anchored in some mythical past. People see the police as constrained by limited resources, and evaluate their detection – and prevention – roles in the light of the unsolvability of many crimes, the prioritization of offences, the volume of calls on police time, and the inability of any system to deter those who are determined to commit crime. Crucially, it emerges that public evaluations of the police are *not* directly centred around crime (see further, Chapter 3). Public expectations of the police – what people want the police for as opposed to what they do not expect them to be able to achieve – are most clearly seen in relation to attitudes toward policing by means of foot patrols, to which we now turn.

## PUBLIC DEMANDS OF THE POLICE: FOOT PATROLS

Much of the debate about general policing methods over the last two decades has been a dialogue between the respective merits of patrolling by car or by foot. Today in England and Wales, most people understand policing to involve car patrols and will only rarely, if ever, encounter an officer on foot. Conventional wisdom, both within and outside the police, has it that the emphasis upon cars has been a mistake and that there should be a switch of resources towards foot patrols. Indeed, a promise embedded in official representations of NW is the restoration of local, community-based officers who will carry out many of their duties on foot. It is well established that people are generally in favour of foot patrols, though there is no systematic information on why foot patrols are valued. In this and the next two sections we examine public attitudes to officers patrolling on foot but, before doing so, it is important to say a little about the history of public attitudes towards car patrols.

### Car patrols

The concept of 'unit beat policing', in which officers patrol by car and are linked to the station by car and personal radio, was introduced in the late 1960s, and modelled on a policing scheme in Kirkby, Lancashire (see generally, Weatheritt, 1986). Though it was never evaluated, the Kirkby scheme was promoted by the police as a success (St Johnson, 1978), and the Home Office encouraged additional expenditure on cars and personal radios (Home Office, 1967a). The official objectives were, among other things, to increase police efficiency, to improve police–public relations, and to increase the accessibility of the police and thereby improve the flow of information to them from the public. So far as the Home Office was concerned, foot patrolling had not been effective in creating good police–public relations (Weatheritt,

1986). Thus, a police training film introducing unit beat policing commented on traditional methods and their replacement in these terms:

> The fine reputation of the British policeman has always stemmed from his being the trusted guardian of law and order. Essentially, this trust has depended on the community feeling that a particular constable belongs to them. Living amongst them for a long period, they know him personally and willingly cooperate with him in his work. Knowing him as their constable, they confide in him and provide him with the information he needs to anticipate and prevent crime.
>
> In the centre of modern towns and cities, this cooperation between public and police has been lost to a considerable degree. In contrast to the village policeman, the town centre policeman finds little opportunity to get to know members of the public. The majority of his time is entirely non-productive in terms of crime detection and of virtually no value in terms of crime prevention. His role is mainly a passive one and what action he does take is often too far removed from the prime concern of the police – the war against crime. This lack of the right communication between public and police leads inevitably to a sense of frustration in both, the former because crime incidence continues to increase and the latter because they cannot obtain sufficient cooperation to take effective action.
>
> (cited in Weatheritt, 1986, p. 92)

Too much must not be made of official rhetoric because, as Weatheritt (1986) points out, the real case against foot patrols in the 1960s was economic: the shortage of officers forced the Home Office into maximizing the area covered by those who were available.

Despite the general approval which greeted its introduction (Martin and Wilson, 1967; Banton, 1973), unit beat policing soon fell into disfavour. When the rise in fuel prices in the mid-1970s and the boom in recruitment of the early 1980s took away the economic imperatives which had led to its proliferation, a new understanding was promoted which attacked the very theory of unit patrol. In the new wisdom, the technologies of the car and the personal radio set up a metal barrier between the police and the public, reducing the opportunities for informal and personal interactions. Removed from the public, officers were said to have lost interpersonal skills and, because of the psychological effects of extended periods of boredom interspersed with occasional moments of tension, to act more abrasively and officiously when incidents occurred (Baldwin and Kinsey, 1982; Manwaring-White, 1983).

Although the technological imperative is widely said to have changed the methods of policing and the values which underlie policing (Alderson, 1979), aspects of car patrols are highly valued by the public. We found, as has other research (Jones et al., 1986), that the public require a fast response when they dial 999. The police were praised on the basis that 'they came quickly when we rang', and criticized if they took what was judged to be a long time in responding. But people distinguished between fast response, which was viewed positively, and car patrols, which were generally viewed negatively. Whilst the two may be linked in practice by the uneven demand on patrolling relief officers, residents saw response as quite distinct from cars 'cruising' around the area and were almost universally against the latter.

Although there is evidence that car patrol officers in general act calmly, sympathetically and authoritatively in dealing with incidents (Ekblom and Heal, 1982), there is little positive sentiment towards car patrolling from the public. The little that there is, as in the following view from a Gwent rural resident, tends to be restricted to areas of scattered population where foot patrolling is seen to be impractical:

> Patrolling in cars is a good thing. It's not alienated people, and there's no way the bobby on the beat can do the job. The bobby on the beat is not needed: what is needed is for someone to drive round here occasionally.

In general, however, policing by car is not favoured by the public who want instead to see a marked increased in patrolling by foot.

## Foot patrols: the general response

It is now well established from research that there is strong public sentiment in favour of foot patrols. Surveys by the Policy Studies Institute (1983) and Hibberd (1985) in London, Kinsey (1984) in Liverpool, and Moss and Bucknall (1982) in Northamptonshire, all report substantial majorities of the public in favour of more foot patrols. A Harris Research Centre survey in 1990, commissioned by the Association of Chief Police Officers, the Police Superintendents' Association and the Police Federation, found that most people thought there were too few police officers around, and most people, especially those in inner city areas, wanted more officers on foot (*Guardian*, 9 March 1990). Broadly similar sentiments can be found in the United States of America (Skolnick and Bayley, 1986). Our findings reinforce these earlier studies, with the overwhelming majority of residents strongly favouring foot to car patrols. Our research provides important new information about why the public favour foot patrols and it is this aspect of our research which we wish to concentrate upon here.

In this section we deal with the *general* response to foot patrol by the public; in the next, we deal with the responses distinctive to the inner city areas. A very small group of residents favour foot patrols because of their assumed crime deterrent value. There were two strands of thought here. Some residents reasoned that foot patrols would make the police more accessible, increase public confidence in the police, and thus lead to the public providing the police with more information about crime and criminals in the community. Others simply assumed that foot patrol officers would see more incidents than those in cars driving at speed through the community. Some examples of these ways of thinking are set out below:

> I'd certainly like to see more of the old-fashioned beat man coming round. They pick up facts and information from people who wouldn't normally bother.

> Local bobbies, I really do think that's the answer. Forget the cars and the whizzing around and that . . . they need to be out walking. They might not see anything but might actually get the community on his side slowly but surely. People at the moment, people in general are very reluctant to go to the police to report anything that's happened anyway because there's too much of it, they don't think anything'll be done. But if you know someone on a first-name basis you're more likely to go to them and say 'Oh, there mightn't be anything in it but somebody's been round the last couple of nights, doing whatever . . .', but you're unlikely to go and do that to a complete stranger, you know, with 'Excuse me officer . . .'.

> I think policing would be more beneficial if we had the bobby

on the beat rather than in the panda car. In the panda car, he passes through here and when he's passed through he's been and gone within a minute. You can't tell me that a man driving a car can see everything that's going on around that particular vehicle when he's proceeding at twenty or thirty miles per hour, up the road, because he just won't: his concentration will be on the driving, not the policing of the area.

The beliefs of this admittedly small group find little support in the research literature. In the United States of America, for example, the Newark foot patrol experiment did not lead to any decrease in the incidence of crime (Police Foundation, 1981). Similarly, in England, Weatheritt's reanalysis of internal police data arising out of a series of foot patrol experiments run by the West Midlands Police in 1981, found that recorded crime *increased* in all the test areas over the course of the experiment (Weatheritt, 1986; West Midlands Police, 1982). It needs to be stressed that the English comparisons have been poorly implemented, with officers unclear about their new objectives or unwilling to carry them out; in the West Midlands Police experiment, for example, one shift had to be abandoned because of the unpopularity of the new arrangements. It follows, therefore, that no clear answer is yet available on the comparative efficiency of foot and car patrols in relation to crime prevention. None the less, there are good reasons for believing that the impact of foot patrols on crime prevention is likely to be slight, as Weatheritt points out:

Aggregate crime figures may look large but, in relation to time and space, criminal acts are relatively rare events. Their rarity means that they are not readily susceptible of being discovered by routine patrols which, because of the amount of ground they have to cover, are bound to be sparse and intermittent. The likelihood of a patrolling officer coming across a crime in progress is slight.

(1986, p. 15)

This perception of the crime value of foot patrols was shared by many people in our survey of residents, as the following illustrative quotations show:

I don't think [walking the beat] does help on crime. If they do walk all day, they just walk. Crimes don't happen all the time; sometimes it does happen, but not all the time.

There's a couple of bobbies around but they are not likely to be in the right place at the right time.

The vast majority of residents, however, want foot patrols for reasons which are *not* directly connected with crime. So far as most people are concerned, officers in cars are unapproachable, inaccessible and detached from the local community. The set of demands made by residents is not simply concerned with officers in cars; it is more generally about the remoteness of policing from the people. Residents persistently told us that they wanted an officer who was *known* to the community and, preferably, someone who *lived* in the community. This was true not only in the big city police areas, but also in the villages in the rural areas where people felt that policing was becoming more detached from the community. In the Gwent rural areas, for example, whilst people were strongly supportive of their police, many people felt that organizational and bureaucratic imperatives were gradually unhooking officers from their beat areas; and in one area it was a source of puzzlement why their 'local' police house was occupied by an officer who worked elsewhere. The demand for local officers was, it must be said again, a demand throughout all force areas:

> I'd like to see them just strolling the streets . . . I have a friend who lives a few miles away and they have a policeman who'll knock on his door and say 'How's things?'. That never happens here.

> I believe in community policing. A policeman should know the community, have a good relationship with the people he serves in the area. They go past in the car and he doesn't know anyone.

For some people, putting officers back on the beat would create or recreate interpersonal skills. There was a strong sense that officers did not know how to communicate with people, a skill-deficit that was not assisted by travelling in a car, 'cut-off' from the general public:

> You want to see more old police. If you want to see [police attitudes] change then you want to see less police in cars where they're impersonal and are threatening. You want to see them out on the streets getting to know people. Even if you only say 'hello'.

> A lot of the younger [officers] don't really know anything about

public relations. Perhaps putting them back on the beat would help achieve it. A good officer is someone who can communicate; that's what it's really all about. Someone who can talk to people, explain to people. You can go to them and ask them, and they can tell you who to apply to and where to go.

It is clear, therefore, that the demands made by the public are essentially symbolic rather than instrumental. People do not generally demand police action: rather, they want police presence to be in a form which makes officers approachable. When pressed as to why they wanted approachable officers, people usually said that this form of policing was reassuring ('Foot patrols are visible and that's reassuring to people'; 'To have someone walking would give a lot more assurance than anyone in a car'). Reassurance, in this context, means no more than that police officers by their presence confirm the stability of social order, doubts about which are implanted with every sensationalized media representation of crime and disorder. This is especially important at times of moral panics, and its value is often recognized by beat officers themselves (the beat officer's presence 'does reassure a public that is becoming increasingly paranoid over what they perceive as a breakdown in law and order': Sgt Greaney, *Guardian*, letters, 4 October 1989).

The demands upon the police are entirely consistent with the subordinate position that crime and fear of crime occupy in the lives of most people (see Chapter 3). People want the barrier between them and the police broken down so that they can enjoy the feeling of comfort and security in personal relations which friendliness brings. This is apparent to community beat officers themselves, who described their dealings with people in personal rather than in crime terms, and who recognized the importance of their symbolic role. The following quotations from community beat officers document how the vital features of social relations are not connected to dramatic and unusual events but rather are firmly anchored in the mundane and routine realities of social exchange:

Q: What are the concerns of people on your beat?
A: Certainly, to some degree, just to know you're there. They really are reassured if they see you walking up and down the street. Quite often people come up and say how nice it is to see a policeman walking the streets.

I spend most of my time wandering, talking to people and making myself available for people to come over and talk to me. Half the time really it's nothing to do with police work, but it is just keeping people happy. They see a policeman on the streets and they feel secure. And that I think is one of the major parts of my job.

I think a lot of the concerns of people are very minor. If they have any, they are very minor. You know: 'A cat got into my garden today, what can you do about it?', very trivial. A lot of people, especially old people, want to speak to me because of loneliness. They've got nothing to make contact with so they make anything an issue. . . . They like to have somebody they know, not just any old police officer. It's trust. They like to see me around. A lot of people do complain that they haven't seen a policeman for two years and things like that. It's reassurance.

Although there is obviously in these remarks a tension between police and public understandings of what the police should be doing ('it's nothing to do with police work', 'it's trivial'), none the less the minimalist demands made by the public are all too clear to the beat officer. Throughout all force areas, the demand for foot patrols was founded in a conception of the police as accessible and approachable. Officers living in and known to the community offered stability and reassurance to people whose background concerns were not centrally concerned with crime.

## Patrolling the inner city: aggressive policing

Whilst there is universal approbation for foot patrols and whilst people express their demand in low-key, personal, and essentially symbolic terms, there is a marked change of emphasis in the inner-city areas of London and Bristol. In these settings the public concern is not about under-policing but about over-policing. Significant aspects of the police – their manner, style, tactics, policies, composition and values – are presented by people as part of the problem of urban existence rather than as part of the solution. The sentiments expressed, the images called up, the rhetoric employed together represent sections of the police force, but not all of it, as external to, and out of step with the needs and demands of the community. People's concerns are not expressed in terms of crime or the area, but in terms of the kind of policing which is imposed on them from outside. This picture emerges in a variety of ways as we shall now document.

The first thing apparent to an observer is that residents of the inner-city areas of London and Bristol think of sections of the police as aggressive and antagonistic towards the local community. This characterization is shared by both white and black people, young and old, male and female. People describe the police as 'threatening', 'aggressive', 'intimidating' and 'hostile'. Where residents in other areas might suggest that some officers lack interpersonal skills, inner-city residents see the police as rude and abrasive, with a predilection for violent confrontation:

> It's quite obvious that people that are recruited into the police aren't recruited for their academic achievements, and very often this kind of prejudice and violence that they're supposed to be policing is prevalent in their own ranks, so that's a kind of paradox.

> How many see it as a branch of the army, a place to go and have a hell of a good time and where ... you can hit your fellow men over the head with impunity because the chances are you can get away with it.

> I think the problems are the same throughout the Met. I think they are a bunch of gangsters really: I mean, that organised and that criminal. . . . I mean they do keep the peace, but it's peace on their terms. . . . I mean you can't pretend that I would be happier if they disappeared, but I am not happy with the way they work at all.

As the last-quoted resident makes clear, these criticisms of the police come from people who said that they favoured law and order and would welcome foot patrols or other non-confrontational policing styles. What then makes people who want to support the police feel so negatively about the policing actually delivered in these two force areas?

The first thing that is apparent from inner-city residents' interviews is that more people spontaneously mention negative encounters with the police than is the case with rural residents. The heavier concentration of police in urban areas increases the likelihood of an encounter, and specific practices of the police, such as stop and search, are engaged in more frequently in the inner city than in suburban and rural areas. Residents regarded the frequency of such encounters and the manner in which they are carried out as provocative:

*Metropolitan resident*
I don't have a lot of faith in the police as they operate at the moment. Like, for example, walking down the street you can get pulled up for something, 'acting suspiciously' or something, when you haven't actually done anything at all. People I know are pulled up regularly every week and they've never been proved to have done anything and they certainly haven't done anything. It's a very difficult issue the police, because we need to have them but not the way they are at the moment.

*Avon and Somerset resident*
I used to get stopped all the time walking home after the pubs had closed. I'd be guaranteed to be stopped literally and have me pockets run through. I've always said: 'Is it gonna be more hassle for me now if I empty my pockets here or if you take me to the station?'. They'd say 'wherever' and I'd say 'well, you can search me now then'. I'd rather that than take me down to the station and give me a load of shit because of my attitude.

*Metropolitan resident*
I was stopped on the road and the police were very aggressive towards me and gave me the whole suspicion thing about why I'd been in this particular shop, and like the whole suspicion that maybe I'd gone to buy drugs there. I was really adamant, I was with a friend, and they were just really arrogant and I really felt for the black youths, eighteen-year-olds hanging on the streets; no wonder, I can imagine what sort of treatment they get. . . . I left feeling furious. So, often I think they can be quite provocative in the way they deal with people.

These responses typify the attitude of residents that policing practices were 'unnecessary', 'heavy' and 'intimidating', a conclusion which is perhaps not surprising given the fact the overwhelming majority of these encounters are non-productive in crime terms (see Willis, 1983; Skogan, 1990) and the fact that some officers in urban areas exhibit a desire for confrontation and 'winding people up' in order to create more explosive situations (Foster, 1989). The perception of residents that urban policing styles are unnecessarily provocative is supported by Foster's observational study of police in London where she found that in one station officers acted in an 'aggressive and sarcastic manner' hoping that those stopped 'would rise to the bait' (ibid., p. 133). It is also supported by the fact that some 10 per cent of arrests arising out of official stop-searches have nothing to do with the 'suspicion' which allegedly underpinned the stop but instead result from a reaction to negatively-viewed police behaviour (see Home Office *Statistical Bulletin*, published quarterly).

Behind these responses, however, lay a bigger source of dispute. Although residents were critical of stop and search practices in general and regarded the police as unsympathetic and aggressive, much of the hostility was directed against a particular form of policing – patrolling in vans. These mobile support units (Territorial Support Groups, District Support Units and the like), the successors of the much-feared Special Patrol Groups (SPG) and Police Support Units (PSU), possess their own command structures and have 'a mandate to assist hard-pressed divisions with particular "high-crime" problems, either through providing additional, preventive patrols or, where necessary, "saturation" policing' (Jefferson, 1990, p. 3). Forged in the crucible of industrial protests, anti-racist demonstrations and public disorders, these units utilize officers seconded for tours of duty who are provided specialist public order training; this enables the police to deliver a paramilitary response in selected situations and locations, and against selected groups of the population.

These support units are a systemic feature of policing in two of the research sites. Police vans or 'carriers', protected by metal grilles and carrying ten or more uniformed officers, are frequently deployed in inner-city areas of both London and Bristol. Sometimes they are stationed in a side road, parked at the roadside, or they may slowly 'cruise' an area. People in both cities regarded these vans with anathema. Indeed, in our interviews, two-thirds of Bristol inner-city residents and some four out of ten of those in London spontaneously criticized police use of patrol vans. For residents, vans created an air of menace and symbolized an abrasive policing style that was spoken of in terms of fear (see also Kettle and Hodges, 1982). What must be understood about this system of policing is that it can be deployed precisely in order to instil such fear: when a bottle is thrown at beat officers or at a patrol car in St Paul's, Bristol, 'we usually drive a task force van through soon afterwards', a Chief Inspector of Avon and Somerset police is reported to have said (*The Independent*, 28 April 1990. See also

Jefferson, 1990, p. 8). The point is not lost on residents of all backgrounds, as the following extended comments from Avon and Somerset inner-city residents make clear:

> I don't think the vans are a good idea at all. It produces a negative response. I know of people who have been walking along and something's happened and they've been jumped on and handcuffed. Nothing's been said to them other than 'Get in the van'. They've been taken to the station and later released and not charged. They've been given an explanation afterwards, but it's a bit off.

> I have got some respect for the law but it's really weird; the only time I feel uncomfortable in this area is when there's a copper about. If I'm walking down [x] Road, I can feel intimidated by the people down there if I let myself be intimidated. But if I walk into St Paul's and there's a meat wagon at the end of the road, which quite often there is, I'm more paranoid about those officers jumping out, giving me the one-two, because I've seen them; I've seen people walk along the road, coppers jump out of a van, grab somebody, a swift kicking, van pulls up, carted into the back and they drive off and life goes on!

> There's nothing more annoying than walking along the road and you can actually feel somebody looking at you, there's a car slowing down behind you and you think 'Am I gonna get beat up here by a gang of thugs or what?' and you turn round and you realise that the thugs are four uniforms standing there. And they're blatantly making you look out of place, they're making you look paranoid, and that's wrong.

> Round here, the only time you come across the police is in force; this area is swamped. It's very antagonistic to be walking along and you've got about fifteen policemen in a van all staring at you.

> You quite often see them driving around in big riot vans but personally that doesn't make me feel any safer.

> I'd quite like to see just more community policing rather than such a heavy police presence when something is going wrong. They would seem less threatening. . . . I think probably they swamp the area compared to the level of crime. They usually just whizz round in patrol cars or riot vans.

Exactly these sentiments were repeated in London, where people in the community called up the same images and recounted similar experiences, with strikingly similar consequences:

> The police do patrol, but not only that, I have occasionally seen bloody great vans: I can't understand what they are up to there; I find that very intimidating, the idea of a whole bunch of policemen just sitting there waiting. They might just seize any old opportunity to, well they must be getting frustrated all sitting in that van, I don't think it's the right way to go about things. I know sometimes they have to do 'swamp' things but I am suspicious: I don't know what they are doing, who are these guys sitting in a van – I do find it intimidating.

> If you're standing in Brixton and a police van full of policemen drives by it's fucking annoying. For what? It'd be better if they all got out and walked around rather than driving by and leering at people.

> I haven't given a great deal of thought to foot patrols. That kind of presence seems safer to me than the kind of presence I've occasionally experienced which is vans going round at night full of policemen. There's a feeling that I'm living in a frightening place I suppose.

> I have had an experience where one night we were coming back down [x] Hill and I could see behind me a police van going like the clappers. So I kept on the inside so it could pass and as it got closer its flashing light went off and it came and followed the car. Eventually it stopped us. There were twelve of them in it, there were three of us in my little car. They got out and they were ready for World War Three. They stopped me because I was showing 'undue caution, undue awareness of the presence of a police vehicle behind me'. I said 'well, what's the purpose of having a blue flashing light and going at about 193 m.p.h. if I'm not meant to be aware of you?'. They were obviously on their way to a big kind of punch up, weren't they, and it got called off, and they just happened to follow the car because they could see me driving within the speed limit. Literally, that's what it was. That's just a typical lot. There's a lot of boys, all psyched up. They want action and there is none, so they stop a car.

*Out of step*

This was not, however, just another kind of policing, more remote, more abrasive and more keenly felt by residents. In both Bristol and London residents of all racial and ethnic groupings were agreed that this policing system was targeted primarily against black people, who, it was believed, bore the brunt of discriminatory policing. In these areas, saying 'being out of step with the community' was usually a coded way of talking about unfair treatment of black people, and a prelude to accounts of racist behaviour witnessed or heard about, often giving rise to demands for more black police officers or other systemic organizational changes to the police. Positive contacts with the police by whites were explained away on the basis that this was expected treatment of whites: 'When I've come into contact, I've never had any problems, although there are very good reasons for that in that I'm white, and articulate.' In negative contacts, whites assumed that if they had been black they would have been treated much worse: 'When I've been suspected of being on the wrong side of the [law], then they haven't been very pleasant at all. I'm sure that's not absolutely typical, but for people who are routinely in this sort of situation, like young blacks, it must be very unpleasant'; 'It reflects my general sense that I would not like to be young and black around here.'

Whereas their own contacts with the police were sometimes described by whites as 'sympathetic', 'polite', and 'deferential', police contacts with black people were described by white residents as 'aggressive', 'unpleasant' and 'provocative'. For their part, black people pointed to the lack of faith in the police among young black people in particular, 'racial harassment' by the police, bad 'attitude', the 'disease of racism', and the endemic nature of the discriminatory practices. Attitudes were felt to be deeply-embedded and whilst black people, as well as their white counterparts, spoke of the need for the ethnic composition of the police to reflect that of the communities served, there was little optimism for short-term change. Our study supports the findings of the third British Crime Survey that the policing of inner-city areas, and the street enforcement patterns of police practices, 'seem to have widened the gulf between ethnic minorities and the police' (Skogan, 1990, p. 43).

## CONCLUSION

The contradictory nature of policing is apparent to people in the community and informs the judgements they make about the police. At one level, people would rather not see the police because police presence is associated with trouble of some kind in the community, but at another level the overwhelming majority of people look to the police to handle trouble of all kinds. People are thus, as one London resident put it, 'in a cleft stick. That's the trouble you see: one doesn't really want them but at time of need then you do want them.' Underlying all appraisals of the police, therefore, is a broad commitment to the principles of law, order and justice, and a general sentiment which is disposed to place trust in a public institution. Public criticisms of the police are, therefore, about changes to the police, not in any sense calls for the abolition of the police. Moreover, in commenting on the police, people offered measured judgements about the sort of service they could realistically expect, given the variety of calls on police time and the resources available to the police.

Against this background, it is clear that there is substantial public concern over the quality of service delivered by the police. Our data matched the findings of national surveys which have uncovered a minority, but growing, dissatisfaction with the police. In most areas, the police were criticized for not patrolling local streets, for not possessing certain interpersonal skills, and for being out of step with the wishes of the local community. Throughout all police areas, there was a clear, almost universal, demand for officers to patrol on foot rather than by car. People do not confuse fast response to 999 calls, which they value, with cruising around neighbourhoods in cars, which has no obvious benefits for them. The primary concern of people is not crime-related and foot patrols offer them what they seek – approachability, accessibility, and symbolic reassurance. This is true of all areas, but overlaying this in the inner cities is a vociferous demand for the abolition of a style of policing that is regarded as confrontational, aggressive, counter-productive and racist. A low-key style of policing with officers living in and representing the communities they serve – the promise of neighbourhood watch – would seem to fit with public conceptions of acceptable policing.

# Chapter 3

# Fear of crime

Although official representations of the sentiments of residents have been couched in terms of 'crime concern' rather than 'fear of crime' in order to avoid suggesting failure on the part of the police to address adequately legitimate demands for security and well-being, in making a public commitment towards crime prevention the police have sought to tap into what they assume to be a large reservoir of public fear of crime. The official assumption has been that citizens are sufficiently worried about the threat of criminal victimization that they will, with limited bureaucratic and organizational support from the police, rally to the defence of their communities by increasing personal security measures and engaging in routine surveillance activity. In this chapter, we examine whether this assumption is well founded; whether citizens think about crime in wholly negative ways; and whether, when they are worried about crime, concern is of a sufficiently high order to stimulate social action on their part.

In popular usage 'fear of crime' is used to convey a range of anxieties about crime from disquiet to terror. People speak, for example, of being given the creeps, scared to death, frightened out of their wits, panic-stricken and paralysed with fear. We have to allow for the fact that the transmission of inner feelings is imperfectly achieved through language and may be unconsciously or deliberately inflated especially in media representations of individual or collective anxieties. Even so, the images constantly evoked do testify to a fear of crime, and that it is a matter of serious social concern. Nor is this concern misplaced. Fear of crime can adversely affect the quality of people's lives in fundamental ways, restricting their freedom to walk in particular localities or at particular times, increasing the cost of social life through personal and household security measures, and, at its worst, inducing a fortress mentality in the home and turning city streets at night into austere and forbidding places by emptying them of people. Fear of crime, then, is a matter of political and sociological importance.

In seeking to measure fear of crime and to explicate its meaning, sociologists have attempted to refine popular usage. There is wide agreement that fear of crime needs to be distinguished from more general concerns about crime as a social problem, and from people's beliefs about crime including its causes, perpetrators, victims and frequency (Furstenberg, 1972; Hough and Mayhew, 1983; Maxfield, 1984). Fear is an emotional and physical response to a perceived threat which involves a 'personalized threat rather than abstract beliefs and attitudes about crime as a problem' (Maxfield, 1984, p. 3). Whilst Garofalo (1981) restricts fear of crime to the sense of danger accompanying the anticipation of physical harm, the better view is that such a restriction fails to give weight to the fact that people can experience deep-seated anxiety about property crimes such as burglary (Hough and Mayhew, 1983, p. 22). Nor need fear be confined to worries about being personally victimized; people may have altruistic worries about crimes being committed against their family and friends.

If there is some agreement on what is to be measured, there is considerable controversy over how fear of crime is best measured. Much of our knowledge of fear of crime is derived from survey work relating to levels of victimization as well as fear of crime, undertaken on a national level by the British Crime Survey (Hough and Mayhew, 1983, 1985; Mayhew *et al.*, 1989) and on a local level in Merseyside (Kinsey, 1985) and Islington (Jones *et al.*, 1986; Crawford *et al.*, 1990), a method which has attracted critical scrutiny (Walklate, 1989). Some of the problems identified, such as where respondents deliberately suppress incidents in their past life, have particular bearing upon whether surveys can adequately measure incidents of victimization, but others are more generalizable in their effect. Thus, for example, the seriousness with which the respondent treats the question and the skill and sensitivity of the interviewer, are factors which have effects in both survey work and methods which employ in-depth interviews. Despite these difficulties, there is general agreement that survey work has increased our knowledge of victimization and of the fear of crime and most discussion, to which we shall return, has focused upon how the data generated should be read (Sim *et al.*, 1987; Brogden *et al.*, 1988).

The method we adopted to explore public conceptions of crime and fear of crime was the in-depth interview. Each interview was conducted on the basis of a standard set of questions, with the interviewer given guided discretion to ask follow-up questions and to probe for further information. Respondents were initially put at ease by questions directed toward their conceptions of the meaning of 'neighbourhood' and whether they felt they were part of a neighbourhood, and of their understanding of 'community' and whether they felt part of any community. Understandings of crime and of fear of crime were then explored in a variety of ways.

First, we sought to discover whether crime was something which figured prominently in their life and in the way they thought about their locality. This was accomplished by an undirected question: what, if any, are the problems for you in this area? Second, we tapped personal concern by asking whether people were willing to walk the local streets after dark, whether people had any concerns about doing so, and whether they had the same feelings about areas other than that in which they lived. The questions related to concern rather than the narrower concept of fear so that we would elicit a broader spectrum of anxieties, and not inhibit people from expressing worries short of fear. Third, we asked whether they considered that crime was one of the problems in their area, thereby seeking to uncover whether they felt crime to be one of several social problems they had, and to prevent them from unconsciously or unthinkingly translating their beliefs about crime generally in the country to their own locality. Fourth, we asked those who identified crime as a problem whether they considered the problem serious. Finally, we reverted to personal anxiety by asking whether the respondent was personally worried or concerned about crime.

Taken together, these different measures helped us to arrive at a broad view of the sense and meaning of crime and fear of crime in the research sites. We would stress again, however, that no method can overcome all potential sampling, definitional and methodological problems involved in exercises of this kind. Thus, whilst we sought in all cases to ensure that interviews were conducted in confidence, in a number of cases partners or parents remained in the room during the interview (and some joined in). The consequence of this, however, would inevitably be a reduction in the reporting of violence *within* the home, especially against women and children. Another limitation of our study is its failure adequately to monitor the extent of fear of crime among the Asian community. The focus upon NW as the principal unit of analysis and the choice of research sites unexpectedly resulted in an inadequate sample of Asian respondents in our citizen survey. This is unfortunate since there is massive under-reporting of racial attacks against Asians; they have a disproportionate likelihood of being victims of crimes such as vandalism and victimization by groups of strangers which cannot be accounted for by demographic and residential factors (Mayhew *et al.*, 1989), and the police have shown a lack of sensitivity towards them (see for example Greater London Council, 1984; Benyon, 1986; Home Office, 1989; Waltham Forest Council, 1990).

In discussing our more general findings on the fear of crime, we shall, at various points, draw upon the findings of other researchers, although it is necessary to point out that strict comparison cannot be made with research using different methods or, as in the Islington Crime Surveys, with research whose methods are not disclosed. And before our findings are discussed it is as well to bear in mind the important point made by Sparks *et al.* that

> we need to be very cautious about interpreting literally expressions of fear of or concern about crime: these may really be expressions of uneasiness about other aspects of experience, or about the state of the world in general.

> (1977, p. 213)

It appears, for example, that isolation, loneliness and lack of community attachment are important sources of fear among the urban elderly (Jaycock, 1978; Yin, 1980; Silverman and Kennedy, 1984). And in our own study, although not seeking to establish direct relationships between such factors and concern about crime, in all our research sites it clearly emerged that people felt little sense of 'community', had a narrow conception of their 'neighbourhood' (often characterized by 'a few houses either side') and were, therefore, insecure in their relationships with 'strangers' in their area, and unsure and suspicious of areas beyond their immediate locale. It seems plausible to conclude, therefore, that some elements of concern about crime simply express uncertain and fractured social relations.

## CONCERN ABOUT CRIME

In common with much other research, we found that crime was a feature of people's thinking in almost all of the areas studied, that concern about crime was significant for some areas and some groups, that most people, irrespective of considerations of possible or likely victimization, engaged in some form of risk-management behaviour, and that for some individuals crime considerations severely affected their life-styles. The threat of crime penetrates every aspect of some people's lives, leading them to install security systems of various degrees of sophistication in the home or car, encouraging some into carrying personal weapons or having these readily available in the home, and leading others into curtailing their activities, typically by avoiding the streets at night.

Concern about crime is evidenced by the fact that large proportions of residents identified crime as a problem of their locality. The lowest ratings were, predictably, in rural areas where fewer than one in eight residents identified crime as a local problem. By contrast, inner-city areas uniformly had a higher rating of crime as a problem, with 75 per cent of inner-city residents in London, 60 per cent in Gwent and 55 per cent in Avon and Somerset identifying crime as a problem of their area. Although crime is commonly understood as a distinctively inner-city phenomenon, we found a less clear-cut picture: two suburban sites (one in Gwent and one in London) exceeded all inner-city areas in terms of the proportion of residents identifying crime as a local problem, and in a majority of suburban sites at least half of the residents interviewed saw crime as a problem of their local area. This general picture is confirmed by the pattern of responses in relation to questions about personal concern over crime.

*Table 3.1* Concern about crime according to location

| Inner-city residents | Suburban residents | Rural residents |
| --- | --- | --- |
| 35.1% | 33.8% | 15.0% |

The following examples illustrate the ways in which residents concerned about crime experienced feelings of anxiety or were moved to change their life-style to accommodate a perceived threat.

*London suburban resident*

Q: Does the crime problem concern you in particular?

A: Yes, I suppose the main concern here is about getting burgled. We haven't got enough money to get insurance so if anything goes it goes, but the stereo is eleven years old, that's rented and its compulsory covered by insurance, that's the only insurance in the house. The only thing is my tools – I am a builder [with] £800–900 worth. If that lot went, then that's my livelihood gone and no insurance to get the tools back. I suppose that's my biggest worry actually.

*London surburban resident*

Q: What are the problems for you in this area?

A: Psychological. Being burgled fifteen times in three years, living behind bars, being mugged. I don't feel happy here.

Q: The unhappiness, is that just because of the fear of crime or other things?

A: It is just crime, because last month I thought I'm beginning to get recognised and that little spark of community/neighbourhood was starting to exist. I was feeling good about that then I came home and got mugged. It's violence and crime. It's completely dark on the stairs when the lights go out. It's dangerous, people lurk and you get mugged on those stairs but you've got to get home.

Q: You mentioned mugging and burglary, do they equally concern you or are there other types of crime?

A: Any infringement of another human being's space or property or possessions is absolutely appalling. After the last burglary I ended up going to see a psychiatrist. Apart from what they've nicked, its what they've touched and seen. You don't know who that person is out on the street; they've seen into you without you knowing who it is. Then getting mugged was even worse. You know your own home isn't safe because that's been violated already and then your body space is violated; the next worst is if you're raped, it's intrusion on a person.

*Avon and Somerset suburban resident*

Q: Can you describe your feelings?

A:   I think as well it is a bit like being a prisoner because you
don't go out, and if you didn't have a car like I have, it would
be horrible because it is so difficult to go out and you are
taking a risk each time you do it. I don't think it matters what
the area is. Obviously in Brixton you are more likely to be
physically attacked there I would think than here, but it's
just a chance isn't it. The odds might be more favourable
[here] but it still doesn't make any difference. I would like
really to see more policemen around, not walking around
hitting people, mainly just so you can feel no need to bother,
you would feel a bit happier walking out. I think it would
make a difference to some of the older people as well; some
I deal with quite a lot in my business, some are very anxious.

*Gwent suburban resident*
Q:   What are the problems, if any, for you in this area?
A:   We are close to the park and one worrying thing is we get a
lot of, well not a lot of, we get break ins. I think it's probably
because we are close to the park, too many people sitting
around idle, without work: they wait their chance and break
in. This is why you'll probably find my house is like a fortress,
bolts, chains, catches on the windows and the dog.

Concern about crime is related not simply to location, but also to
gender and age, though we may note in passing that in the present
study there were no variations in reported levels of crime concern
according to race. Previous research in the United States of America and England, for example, tends to show strongly that women
and the elderly report much higher levels of fear than do others
(Skogan and Maxfield, 1981; Hough and Mayhew, 1985; Kinsey,
1985; Crawford *et al.*, 1990). The Merseyside Crime Survey put
the point clearly in relation to women:

> The picture which has emerged is one of people of the inner
> city – especially the women – living under curfew. While . . . the
> actual chances of victimization are less than many people believe, none the less, in Granby, for example, three quarters of
> those interviewed believe there are real risks for women who go
> out at night and half said they often or always avoid going out
> after dark.
>
> (Kinsey, 1985, pp. 23–4)

In line with this, we found that women reported much higher

levels of personal concern about crime than men, as Table 3.2 shows:

*Table 3.2* Personal concern about crime according to sex

| Men | Women |
|-----|-------|
| 23.3% | 37.3% |

The gendered nature of concern about crime is understandable in view of the under-reporting and under-recording of crimes against women (Chambers and Millar, 1983; Hanmer and Saunders, 1984; Russell, 1984; Stanko, 1984) and the systematic underplaying of violence against women *within* the home (Renvoize, 1982; Stanko, 1988). Feminist writers have only recently begun to explore how women's *everyday* experiences are marked by feelings of insecurity and the likelihood of being a victim of male aggression and violence (Walklate, 1989). This has led Kelly to suggest that the nature of sexual violence should be reconceptualized in terms of a continuum:

> Using this concept of a continuum highlights the fact that all women experience sexual violence at some point in their lives. It enables the linking of the more common, everyday, abuses women experience with the less common experiences labelled as crimes. It is through this connection that women are able to locate their own particular experiences as being examples of sexual violence.
>
> (1987, p. 54)

The gendered construction of fear is supported in our study, where women's concerns were often directly expressed in terms of *men* rather than in terms of crime in general, as the following illustrate:

*Suburban resident*
Q: What sort of person, if any, would arouse your suspicions in this area?
A: Men, and groups.
Q: Any other types of person?
A: No.

*Suburban resident*

Q: What sort of person, if any, would arouse your suspicion in this area?

A: Being a sexist here . . . men.

Q: Why do you say that?

A: Mainly because of their air . . . the fact they have power in themselves.

Q: All men?

A: Yeah, all men have power over women in general. Certainly at night, if I'm walking around on my own or something and there's a guy behind me, then I get uptight.

Q: What do you do in that type of situation?

A: Walk quicker. Walk into a local shop if I really got intimidated by someone . . . that type of thing.

*Inner-city resident*

Q: What, if anything, would make you suspicious?

A: Men. Probably young, not necessarily black or white because the people I've heard of being mugged have been mugged by white people. If a young man was walking towards me at night I'd feel suspicious I suppose. Women, I wouldn't feel suspicious about them at all, even after an incident recently where I saw a mugging done by a gang of girls.

As the comments of this last-quoted respondent indicate, the connection between crime and fear of crime is not linear but is, to an unexplored extent, mediated by gender role expectations. Moreover, care needs to be exercised in over-reading the data on male and female rates of concern about crime because masculinity ideologies lead to under-reporting of concern by men. This is evidenced by two general findings in our study: male concern about crime was most often expressed in terms of an altruistic concern for others, particularly partners; and male denials of concern were usually expressed in terms of their physical ability to deal with any trouble ('I can take care of myself', 'I'm still fit and can handle any trouble', 'I can still take care of myself but in a few years I won't so I'll need a stick or something' were typical responses).

In the literature on concern about crime, it is a commonplace to treat the elderly alongside women. A number of studies have found that both groups report much higher levels of fear than do others (Skogan and Maxfield, 1981; Hough and Mayhew, 1983;

Maxfield, 1984). This had led in the United States to the conclusion that for older people 'fear of crime is even more of a problem than crime itself' (Costa, 1984) and that levels of self-imposed 'house-arrest' among the elderly constitutes a national crisis (Goldsmith and Tomas, 1974). Interestingly, in our research there was no consistent relationship between age and crime concern. Whilst the youngest group were least concerned about crime, greatest concern was expressed by those between the ages of 20 and 40, as Table 3.3 shows:

*Table 3.3* Personal concern about crime according to age and sex

| Age | Proportion of men, % | Proportion of women, % | Overall proportion |
| --- | --- | --- | --- |
| Under 20 | 16.7 | 20.0 | 18.0 |
| 20 to 39 | 23.1 | 43.9 | 33.8 |
| 40 to 59 | 19.0 | 31.6 | 25.0 |
| 60 and over | 28.6 | 30.0 | 29.0 |

Two factors perhaps help explain these patterns. First, as other research has also demonstrated (Jones, 1986) factors other than crime are of greatest concern to elderly people, in particular, health and coming to terms with their mortality. Second, some women reported a reduced fear as they grew older, a finding which may be consistent with the argument of some writers that female concern about crime is a dialogue with anxiety about rape (Riger *et al.*, 1978; see also Maxfield, 1984). The following interview excerpt illustrates this point:

*Suburban resident*
Q: Are you willing to walk the local streets after dark?
A: Yes I do. I do it rather briskly and don't tremendously enjoy it, but I do.
Q: Do you have any concerns about walking the local streets at night?
A: Yes, I certainly wouldn't recommend anyone to walk from the station to here when dark; even if they were male, let alone female.
Q: How do you feel about walking at night in other areas?
A: Well I never used to bother about it very much. In some

ways I don't suppose I do now because I am older and one
is more worried when younger for obvious reasons as a
woman so it is probably about equal. Now I am older I
probably worry less, and when I was younger the streets
were safer but I worried more.

Another factor known to be related to concern about crime is prior
victimization. A victimizing experience may render a person vulnerable, creating a sense of insecurity and uncertainty, and
displacing feelings of confidence and trust. Whilst it may be true
that many victims of even relatively serious offences seem 'able to
cope without significant practical or emotional problems' (Hough
and Mayhew, 1985, p. 52), for some the experience of victimization
can be devastating (Maguire, 1982; Shapland *et al.*, 1985; Maguire
and Corbett, 1987; Mawby and Gill, 1987). Although we did not
systematically examine the issue of prior victimization, the ways in
which people's lives were affected by a prior experience emerged
clearly in our interviews, as in the following examples:

*Inner-city Gwent resident*
Q: Is there a crime problem in this area?
A: Yes. It's definitely increased.
Q: What form does it take?
A: Burglaries mostly. Attacks on cars; came home one day, and
   seven had all had their tyres slashed.
Q: Would you say that these are serious?
A: Yes.
Q: Would you actually say that there is a serious crime problem
   here?
A: Yes.
Q: Do you feel particularly concerned about it?
A: Yes. . . . There's two sixteen year old boys who broke in here,
   who were on the run. I mean sixteen years of age! They
   broke in here, they went through all our things, they took
   the video, we were lucky they caught them, and they
   smashed the windows. When people used to say 'it's awful
   when you have your house broken into, it's not what they
   take, it's the fact that someone's been in the house', I used
   to say 'that's stupid', but that's true; that is because every
   time I used to open that door I used to go cold, it's a horrible
   feeling to know that people have been through all your

things, and through your drawers and through your clothes. We can't open the back window now, it's nailed down.

*Suburban London resident*

Q: Although you say you don't feel part of your neighbourhood, can you tell me what your neighbourhood is exactly?

A: Within these four walls. . . . There is a reason for that. My husband was mugged very recently, and I feel very frightened now to walk out on the streets with my baby. He was threatened with a knife, and his money and belongings were all taken away, but he wasn't injured in any way. . . . I don't go out on the street and walk around with the pram because I'm frightened.

Q: Is this fear with you all the time once you've left your front door?

A: Yes. Not so much during daylight and the morning, but I'm always looking behind me, seeing who's coming, and walking fast if I see some shady character standing on a corner, or whatever. This is more because of the baby, really.

*Suburban London resident* (recently burgled)

Q: Do you think there's a crime problem in this area?

A: To be honest with you, I think there's a crime problem everywhere. There's always a problem when someone like myself gets burgled or attacked or whatever. . . . Last week [before I was burgled], I'd probably have said to you 'I've had no knowledge of a crime problem at all'.

Q: Does the crime problem concern you in any way?

A: Again, last week I would have said no; this week I'd probably say yeah. I mean, this week, the house is belled up, I've got a dog, if someone got in and they got to the bedroom, they'd have some surprises . . . y'know, all these things which I spent a lot of money doing, which I didn't envisage doing really.

Research suggests that the majority of victims of most types of crime recover from the worst psychological effects within a period of a few weeks. However, for a substantial minority of victims of serious violent crime and a smaller proportion of other offences, victimization causes lasting changes in their personality and behaviour (Maguire and Corbett, 1987, pp. 69–70). This variable effect of prior victimization was apparent in our study, with a few respondents reporting long-term effects of prior victimization, as in the following example:

*Rural Gwent resident*

Q: Do you feel personally concerned about crime and the threat of crime here?

A: I think one has a great awareness. I was burgled twice in my other house, my parents' house, and there wasn't a lot to take. I think if one's had that experience, then I think you have an awareness. I think crime's a funny thing. I think they'll catch somebody who's done a crime and they'll punish him because he's pinched a video and something and I think they don't consider the damage it's done to the person who's been the victim, because my mother had a nervous breakdown, and she didn't ever get really well again, and that was the result of a burglary.

Q: How long have you felt the need to be more vigilant than you were.

A: Well, heavens! We had the break in twenty odd years ago, and I should say from then, twenty-five or thirty years ago; this isn't a new thing with me. I think it's been because we had the experience of it and you can't trust anybody really, you don't trust the chap who brings the milk, the chap who comes to mend the electric wire, it's a sad story.

Taken together these findings go some way to supporting the critique levelled against official attitudes to public concern over crime by the new realist criminology. Official pronouncements arising out of analyses of British Crime Survey data have tended to depict fear of crime as, in part at least, an irrational response to likely risks of victimization. Hough and Mayhew, for example, in a much-cited passage, sought to put the risks of victimization into context in the following terms:

a 'statistically average' person aged sixteen or over can expect: a robbery once every five centuries (not attempts), an assault resulting in injury (even if slight) once every century, the family car to be stolen or taken by joyriders once every sixty years, a burglary in the home once every forty years.

(1983, p. 15)

This approach leads to the conclusion that fear of crime is a problem in itself and that better information about the real, rather than imagined, risks of criminal victimization should be provided in order to reduce anxiety about crime.

> People's anxieties might be more realistic if the mundane reality were apprehended – that the majority of burglaries are committed by teenagers; that most offenders will be highly apprehensive about encountering the householders, and being confronted by a burglar is extremely rare; that burglars usually take a small amount of easily disposable goods; and that they will take as short a time as they can, not waiting about to vandalise the home.
>
> (Hough and Mayhew, 1983, p. 27)

On the basis of local surveys, the new realist criminology school has challenged this official line. Uncovering a greater incidence of criminal incidents against women, the poor, and ethnic minorities than was suggested in the British Crime Survey, writers such as Young, Kinsey and Lea have concluded that the perception of risk is often related to relative vulnerability, that fears or concerns about crime are not 'unrealistic' and that for the poor, the weak and the vulnerable 'losing the fight against crime is the worst crime of all' (Kinsey *et al.*, 1986). Instead of educating away people's anxieties, the new realists argue among other things that such fears should be taken seriously, that policing should be re-oriented towards crime and away from order-maintenance, and that there should be a broad, democratic, multi-agency approach (including a modified neighbourhood watch) to crime.

In our view, the conclusions of the new realists, whilst containing elements with which we agree, are profoundly mistaken. We reach our position not only upon the basis of serious doubts about interpretation of their own data (on which, see Brogden *et al.*, 1988, p. 185 ff.) but, more important, upon our assessment of the ways in which people conceptualize crime and give crime meaning and substance in their lived experiences. Whilst we agree with the new realists that people's real concerns, however related to actuarial risks, should not be underplayed, and that fear of crime can produce devastating consequences for certain individuals, none the less our research contests the view that the fear of crime is such a prominent feature in most people's lives. The question is not whether fear of crime should be taken seriously, but how important a part should it play in theorizing about crime and constructing public policy initiatives relating to crime. Our research shows that for the overwhelming majority of people, crime, if it figures at all, is a background consideration of their lives and not the organizing matrix of their normal activities. The reasons which move us to this conclusion now need to be addressed.

## CRIME CONCERN IN CONTEXT

Whilst crime is a matter of concern to many people, concern is quite different from fear. For most people, crime is not an ever-present spectre and, even where it becomes visible or occupies their thoughts, it is not seen in a simple undifferentiated way. For most people, crime in its ordinary representation does not produce images of violence and destruction, even intrusion: it is instead seen as part of the mundane realities of life which will rarely have catastrophic consequences. Problems other than crime dominate the lives of ordinary citizens. When they think about crime, and often when they experience it, crime is seen as episodic and non-serious. Similarly, although images often associated with the perpetrators of crime, and still cultivated in official literature (King, 1989), dwell on various representations of evil and wickedness, most citizens see criminals as ordinary people whose behaviour can be understood even if not excused. We document in the following six sub-sections, how most people come to have a concern about crime rather than a fear of it.

### Non-directed references to crime

One of the central planks of the realist view of fear of crime is the identification of crime as a problem by respondents. In the most recent Islington Crime Survey (Crawford *et al.*, 1990), crime was one of the most serious problems spontaneously cited by respondents, and crime was cited more frequently than other problems (Table 2.2, p. 23). This contrasts with the findings of the second British Crime Survey (Hough and Mayhew, 1985), when respondents were asked to identify the worst things about living in their area:

> Across the country as a whole, 5 per cent mentioned crime and vandalism as the worst aspect. Other problems clearly outweighed crime. Poor amenities and shopping facilities were cited by 13 per cent, traffic was the worst problem for 11 per

cent overall, more in cities; poor transport was cited by 7 per cent, but by more in rural areas. 8 per cent identified signs of social disorder or 'incivilities' – the non-criminal or marginally criminal behaviour of tramps, drunks, rowdy youths, or noisy neighbours.

(Hough and Mayhew, 1985, p. 40)

Our findings correspond with those of Hough and Mayhew and support the early critiques of new realism which pointed out that, even on its own terms, new realist evidence did not support the view that crime was a major fear in people's lives and that unemployment, bad housing and lack of facilities for young people were more important (see Malik, 1986; Sim *et al.* 1987, p. 47). For the most part, crime was not spontaneously mentioned as a problem of the locality even in inner-city areas: and where it was mentioned, it tended to be just one more of the neighbourhood problems. Crime and concern over crime is for most people a latent rather than a manifest issue (see Scheingold, 1990, pp. 192–4). This is shown in the following illustrative responses from residents in inner city areas who were asked to identify the problems for them, if any, in their locality:

*London residents*
Dog shit! Noise, traffic, people speeding, screeching tyres round corners, dogs barking and dog shit really. That is the most immediate thing.

Well, there isn't really a decent shopping centre.

Really noisy. And you have got people playing music, and you have got dogs messing around everywhere, and all around you just keep hearing sound.

The shops are a problem because there is none in the immediate vicinity. I have to travel a fair distance even to do the laundry. I would say being black, but I don't find it a problem.

*Avon and Somerset residents*
The mosque nearby and all their noise. That has been my only problem recently.

For me personally I have no problems directly related to the area.

The dustmen haven't been for ages which really miffs me because there is rubbish absolutely everywhere. That is one problem I can name straight off. Street lighting is improving since I have been here, they have put new ones in, as there were not many down this street at all. I don't really use the buses, they don't seem to publicise where they go, so I have no idea where they go so I tend not to use them.

*Gwent resident*
Unemployment, no place to go at night.

I couldn't specifically pinpoint one thing. I suppose basically it would be down to noise.

For most people, crime is not at the forefront of their social concerns, which tend instead to be dominated by what the police would term 'grief'. Noisy neighbours, kids kicking a ball against the side of their house, unemployment, environmental mess, transport, poor local facilities – these are the stuff of everyday life.

## The seriousness of crime

A second way in which the relegated importance of crime emerges is in the way in which people judge crime as 'serious'. We have indicated already that *concern* about crime is, at some level, a feature of most people's thinking in all areas studied, but it must be understood that this is quite different from *fear* of crime. Although some people can truthfully be said to be fearful of crime – to be frightened of strangers, scared of groups, alarmed at the onset of night and haunted by the prospect of being victimized – to say it of most people would seriously misrepresent their feelings. These instead are characterized more by an awareness of the possibility of crime, and a general sense of avoiding what are felt to be manifestly dangerous situations. In great part, this attitude is founded in people's evaluation of most crime as non-serious. Thus, although a large proportion of people said that crime was one of the local problems, most of those said that it was not a *serious* problem, as Table 3.4, which sets out some representative findings from each force area, illustrates.

*Table 3.4* Seriousness of the crime problem, as expressed by locality

| Residents | Crime is a problem, % | Crime is a serious problem % |
|---|---|---|
| London, inner city | 75.0 | 16.0 |
| London, suburban | 60.0 | 10.0 |
| Gwent, inner city | 60.0 | 30.0 |
| Gwent, suburban | 80.0 | 10.0 |
| Avon and Somerset, inner city | 55.0 | 11.0 |
| Avon and Somerset, suburban | 67.0 | 11.0 |

Those who rated crime as serious did so for a variety of reasons (cf. Rossi *et al.*, 1974; Walker, 1978). For some it was directly related to previous victimization, as in the following example:

*Inner-city resident*
Q: Is there a crime problem in this area?
A: I've been in this area four years and I've been in houses that have been broken into five times. In this house, it's been three attempts and cars have been damaged. And muggings and rape, though that sort of thing has gone down recently.
Q: Would you say that the crime problem is serious?
A: Yes, I think it is quite serious, happening regularly and to people who live in the area, which makes it difficult to have that sense of trust in the neighbourhood.

This was not, however, the typical reason offered. People generally advanced one of three reasons for viewing crime as serious: that all crime was serious; that crime though not serious for them was probably serious for others; and that behaviours linked to crime suggested that crime was serious. For some people, crime of all kinds was deeply anti-social and deserving of condemnation; and, even where they had described crime problems of the area as not impinging on their lives or even as 'petty' or 'minor', when asked whether the crime problem was serious, said that *any* crime was serious. A second group saw crime as a problem for others, particularly women and the elderly, rather than for themselves. As one suburban resident put it:

I would say it was serious. I don't think about it that much: I am aware of it, but it doesn't affect the way I live. But that is because I'm a bloke. I think if I was a woman it would definitely affect the way I lived.

The largest group, however, were people who had been *taught* that local crime was serious. Thus, in the suburban area of London in which the proportion of people rating crime as serious was higher than in any inner-city area, almost all residents gave as their reason the high premiums for household insurance resulting from frequent burglaries. That told residents, as one put it, that 'crime must be a serious problem'. Similarly, in the Gwent inner city area in which almost one-third of residents saw crime as a serious problem (see Table 3.4, above), the seriousness of crime was made apparent by the fact that many people had recently acquired alsatians, dobermans and other large dogs. High insurance premiums and the sudden appearance of large dogs in the locality teach people that crime must be a serious local problem.

For most people, however, crime is not regarded as a serious problem. There were three sets of reasons which were discernible here and we shall say a little about each in turn. First, even where people acknowledged that some activities amounted to criminal behaviour, these were judged to be 'petty' or 'minor' and not as matters of serious social concern.

*Inner-city Gwent resident*
I don't think it's real crime. Of course you always get some of the wilder, young people more or less, they haven't matured yet; I think you get that, but on the whole it is quite good.

*Suburban London resident*
Q: Would you say that there is a crime problem in this area?
A: Yes, burglary, handbag theft, cars get broken into in front of the house.
Q: Would you say that it is a serious problem?
A: It's irritating, it spoils your value of life, it's not frightening, just a niggle.

This sort of response was sometimes accompanied by fairly graphic accounts of incidents which had occurred in the past, and in all areas (even in the inner city) evaluations were often based on comparison with other areas felt to have a more serious problem, as in the following examples drawn from London:

I seldom think about crime, because there is not really a lot to say about it. The only recent incident was a bloke was mugged on the corner and that sounded quite severe and he went off to hospital and there was a lot of blood on the pavement. But that was about two or three weeks ago; but it was the first thing for ages. You hear people arguing and you get the odd fight and things and I think there is a lot of burglary, at least there was at one stage; but I don't think there is any major crime. No more than you would expect with this variety of people living in one area. Inner-city feeling about it, you know?

Q: Would you say there is a crime problem in this area?
A: *Not really no, that is the point*; obviously it's got to be relative but compared to some suburban areas. You go out to Romford and places like that; it's much worse really, more tension. There is much more chance of getting beaten up in Romford or mugged, I would have thought. And the rate of burglaries is probably high as well. I wouldn't know, but I would guess it would be. (original emphasis)

You could probably think of a good few examples and try and say there is a crime problem. But I think there is more chance at the moment of overreaction to it, I mean there is a little incident happened a few months ago out of the front of the house. You got someone came past and started a fight for no apparent reason, and someone called the police. Within about three minutes there was half a dozen squad cars, a transit van and it was like one fight involving two people and one person trying to break it up. That might be appropriate in some areas where the police themselves might find themselves under attack if they try to do anything, but then again they are going to provoke that reaction by turning up like that. I would say there is more of a problem with people overestimating things than anything else really.

The second group were people who saw (accurately) the main crime problems as relating to property – criminal damage or vandalism to cars, thefts of various kinds, and burglary of dwelling houses – and these were clearly of less concern to them than crimes of violence against the person. And this remained true for many people who had themselves been victims of these kinds of offences; the mundane reality of 'normal' crimes had perhaps helped allay the worst fears which media images of the 'wrecked and desecrated home' variety had inspired. Here are some examples from our three force areas:

*London residents*
The main crime that I am aware of is break-ins, generally kids. I call that sort of petty crime really, people trying to seize an opportunity.

No, I don't consider it serious. Perhaps I don't have the same views on property. I mean, crimes involving violence is what I consider serious – it's not so intrusive and, after all, property is only property.

The people next door have been burgled a couple of times. Not too serious. There isn't a crime problem in the area. I'm not particularly concerned about it.

*Avon and Somerset*
Q: Is there a crime problem in this area?
A: Yes, but not of sort of major proportions. There's an increasing risk of break-ins to your house. This is one of the disadvantages and likelihoods of living in a large, comfortable house. If you live in a large, comfortable house you run the risk of less fortunate or more criminally minded people taking advantage of you. So yes there's risk of break-in and there's apparently a very high risk of having things nicked from the cars. That seems to be the problems that we are having round here. There's minimum street violence. There is street violence but minimal.
Q: Would you say there is a serious problem in this area?
A: No.
Q: Do you feel personally threatened?
A: Not at all.

*Gwent*
I think we get our fair share of break-ins and things like that.... It is not serious. On odd occasions I've spoken to policemen they say we get these small break-ins.

The final group rated crime as not serious on the basis that it did not figure prominently in their lives. Basic security measures were often taken but these were regarded as 'sensible' precautions, undertaken as a matter of course and not unduly impinging on people's thoughts. Simple security steps had become incorporated into people's routines and beyond this it was felt unnecessary to worry about crime or to see crime as serious. The following examples show how people in this group viewed crime as something to be aware of but not as a serious intrusion into their lives:

> You have to check everything is locked up. It's a bit of a pain but it's just a reality.

> [Crime] doesn't really worry me. I do think about it, but if I went round thinking about it all the time, I wouldn't enjoy my life.

> Crime is not what I think of when I leave the house. You know, I'll check the locks and that, but it's more the gas plates on the oven or if I've left the water on.

> We've always been a standard family in that we've locked the doors, locked the windows when we go out. We've always been fairly security minded, but not *over* cautious. (original emphasis)

> I think it's like most areas; you have to be aware of the area you are living. . . . I am not stupid: I don't walk in the back streets, so I suppose I am thinking about it. But I don't walk along wondering when I see someone else walking: but I suppose it's part of the reason why I have never felt threatened.

## Differentiated concern

The third way in which the non-serious evaluation of crime is reached by people, is through their denial of crime as presenting a *general* problem. Although some people believe that crime is a problem, that crime of all kinds is occurring frequently, and that there is a general problem of crime throughout the country, most people are very discriminating in their assessment of crime. This is most apparent in the way in which residents distinguished between crimes and between areas. In respect of the latter, Bottoms *et al.* accurately observed on the basis of a local crime survey that

> adjacent areas . . . can appear . . . to be very similar and can even be almost identical demographically . . . yet they can have very different crime rates, and can be perceived by their residents as presenting very different levels of social problems.

> (1987, p. 151)

Our findings support these observations, with residents persistently drawing distinctions between roads that were, to an outsider, identical, and between crimes which were or were not of concern to them. This was a common response from residents – across all the research sites – and supports the findings of American research which show that substantial proportions of people avoid going into certain areas of the city at night or even during the day (Kelling *et al.*, 1974; Garofalo, 1977; Institute for Social Research, 1975). The following quotations illustrate the area and offence discriminations people made:

> I'm not particularly concerned because I realise anyone can be a victim of crime. It depends what kind of crime you're talking about. Violent crime, I don't believe my chances of being attacked are that great in this area. Mugging, again I don't think so. Burglary is something else, it will eventually happen to everybody to some degree; it happened at my Mum's house when I was a lot younger.

> I wouldn't have thought there is a great deal of crime here. You see burglaries now and then, but nothing out of hand. The car has been sitting outside there for over a year and hasn't had anything done to it. There are a few break-ins to cars around here.

> We are not afraid to live here, but in the next road down in the Crescent that's where they get most of the burglaries: it is quite a regular thing, at least every twelve months if not more.

> Burglary is the most important local crime. . . . I haven't actually heard of any assault or anything like that, more serious crimes, in the actual road itself. I mean, one hears about incidents in [an adjacent city area], stabbings and muggings and so on, but within this road those serious sorts of crimes haven't happened. It's mainly theft.

## Episodic concern

Although concern about crime is sometimes depicted as an all-pervading, endemic feature of life, particularly in city areas, the reality is that it is far from constant. Nor should there be any surprise about this. Official and media representations of crime often talk about 'crime waves', a 'spate of crime', an 'outbreak of burglary' and other similar terms. Crime can be made a more immediate concern by such images or by those picked up from friends and neighbours retelling experiences or rumours. Without such knowledge or rumour transmission, crime may recede into insignificance. Moreover, it is well established that neighbour-hoods can move from high- to low-crime status within relatively short time spans (Kobrin and Schuerman, 1981). Crime is shifting and people incorporate this into the way they address crime concern:

> There was [a crime problem] a couple of years back, quite a few break-ins around here, but we didn't suffer from that. . . . There was a spate of break-ins, but that's all. I wouldn't go so far as to say there was a crime problem; it just happened in a short period, then they were finished with.

> I was more aware of crime when we came here ten years ago: a friend of mine was mugged quite savagely and we were burgled three times when this place was being refurbished.

> There is not a crime problem as far as I know. . . . You may get a run of it and then you may hear of it once, and then nothing.

> What I'm prepared to do depends, like if I had heard of someone being recently attacked then it would make me more cautious about going out or if there is a little bit of unrest in St Paul's you get a bit more cautious about going out.

## Crime tolerance

Official and media accounts of crime paint it as black as possible, dwelling upon those offences which cause most physical and property damage, and those which inflict most distress. Such offences, as the British Crime Survey and other research shows, tend to be unusual, with most crimes not involving great social damage. Many people do not regard certain offences as 'criminal' or as ones about which they should respond negatively. Moreover, and particularly in urban areas, people have come to accept a certain level of crime as part of their 'natural' environment. For these people, there is no reason to view routine occurrences which do not disturb their well-being as matters of serious social concern. Views of these kinds can be seen in the following quotations:

*Inner-city Avon and Somerset resident*
[This white middle-aged woman said that crime was not a problem in her area. She was then pressed on specific crimes which were said to be current in the locality]
Q: Is graffiti a problem?
A: Mostly people who are unemployed do that. Something to do, they are very good at it. Brilliant, it looks really nice. They spray it and its not very easy to do. At least they do that to pass the time rather than murdering people and robbing them.
Q: Is there a drugs problem?
A: The Rastafarians believe that herbs are grown on this earth to be smoked and that is what they believe. If someone comes up to you and asks you if you want drugs, they are not forcing you, I mean it is your own decision. Not this area, but if you go up to St Pauls, you can see them selling it. They are not pushy with a knife at your throat.

*Inner-city Gwent resident*
Q: Would you say that there's a crime problem in this area?
A: No. There's plenty of crime, there's no problem.
Q: What sort of things?
A: Anything they can deal in they get. They steal it.
Q: Would you say that it's quite a serious problem here?
A: No. It's like I said everybody keeps themselves to themselves. Everybody smokes so everybody's the same. When a fight does start, it's usually gang fights.

Whilst these sorts of comment were among the more overt in their toleration or condonation of some crimes, it was very common to encounter people passing off crime as not important on the basis that it was 'part and parcel of life, so you don't notice it any more' (suburban London resident) and that there would be no justification for taking it too seriously: 'Let's face it, people are going to break into houses, aren't they? That's going to happen whatever' (suburban London resident).

## The political dimension to crime

A consistent and somewhat surprising theme to emerge in our interviews was the way in which people's perception of crime was mediated through their recognition of the 'political' dimension of crime. Only in very exceptional instances, as in the following example, did we encounter anyone who attributed crime or the 'rise in crime' to a general 'moral' decline, a drop in standards of social behaviour:

> I think the moral standards of the country as a whole, over the last forty–fifty years have declined. The question of theft, I think there is a lot more of. I don't attribute it in any way to the present political situation, because I think back to 1930 when this country was in a pretty poor way, there was vast unemployment, but you didn't have the same amount of theft and crime. I think there's something radically wrong, whether it stems from the fact that the church is no longer a feature in people's lives, it's difficult to say. Discipline, all kinds of things.

Instead, crime and poverty are inextricably linked in people's minds. The findings of critical criminology over the past forty years – that crime is prevalent throughout the class structure and that the social costs of corporate illegalities far exceed those of lower-class criminals (Pearce, 1973; Reiman, 1979; Box, 1981; Clarke, 1990) – do not appear to have penetrated the world-view held by most people. Instead, people link crime to social justice, poverty, deprivation and unemployment.

This linkage has profound effects upon the way people think about crime and upon the way they think about offenders. In particular, the more people attribute crime to or associate it with poverty, unemployment and inequalities of wealth, the more they shift the focus of concern away from stereotypical images of the 'violent stranger' and 'the outlaw of society' and instead towards the wider political dimension. This has the effect both of causing people to view offenders more sympathetically – characterizing them as themselves victims of a wider order – and also of downgrading any fear they might otherwise have entertained by seeing crime as committed by ordinary people who inhabit their own or adjacent localities.

A second and related effect is to reduce the tendency to blame, by diffusing responsibility for crime to broader societal considerations, thereby implicating people in general in the responsibility for law and order. A third effect is to encourage in people the view that crime problems are related to deep structural and long-term issues which cannot be appropriately addressed by 'instant' or short-term measures, including neighbourhood watch. The following quotations demonstrate these viewpoints:

*Suburban resident*
I'm not politically minded, one way or the other really, so there's Labour saying that it is, there's the Tories saying we're doing something about it, you know – who do you believe?

I mean, I suppose that as people become more and more poor, they will turn to crime. I mean, there's no doubt that if I got desperate, I would do something like that, and the more you need, the more you'll go that way, basically.

*Suburban resident*
On a philosophical level I think it's down to things like unemployment and education and all those bigger things. . . . Statistics don't prove anything as far as I'm concerned. If you're walking down the road and you haven't got any money and you haven't got a job and you see someone who's got something . . . you feel pissed off about it. I mean, I can't agree with it as an action but I can understand what happens.

*Inner-city resident*
Q: Would you like to see a neighbourhood watch scheme set up here?
A: I don't think it would make any difference. . . .
Q: How does the idea of meeting with the police and discussing the problems of the area strike you? Would you be prepared to do that?
A: Not really because at the moment the police are working under a Conservative government that believes that in areas like this the problems are down to the people. They don't recognise the fact that in a depressed area, crime becomes an alternative. So you'd be talking to people that see the problem from a totally different angle; so I don't think we'd have much to say to each other.

*Inner-city resident*
The problems in this area are homelessness and people suffering at the lower end of the class structure from the way the government treats people. I think the government are out for supporting the middle classes and people who are doing alright and they get encouraged because the government says that anybody with enterprise deserves to get rewarded. That's fine

but not everyone has the bottle to do it, so I sympathize with those people.

*Suburban resident (recent burglary victim)*
Q: Does the crime problem concern you, in particular?
A: I think I'm more annoyed than worried. I'm very concerned about *why* there is a crime problem, probably more concerned about the causes than I am about the effects. Because we're all insured up to the hilt, who cares about the video...? There's obviously got to be a lot more done in the way of prevention and education, and there's much greater need for more general political awareness about these deeper problems. It's increasingly becoming a case of the have's and the have-not's, where property attracts crime.

Time and time again, residents sought to make sense of a world in which criminal offences were apparent by seeing a direct connection between criminal behaviour and social deprivation. This social construction of reality was most evident in middle-class neighbourhoods, where sympathy toward criminals and tenderness in terms of remedies for crime might be less expected than in areas which were themselves at the poor end of the social scale. The link between crime and political economy, so assiduously contested by politicians but now receiving powerful support from official Home Office researchers (see Field, 1990), is, according to our survey, readily embraced by sections of property-owning middle classes. For this group, crime is a world in which 'underprivileged people [are] trying to grab something for themselves', where the divide between the propertied and the propertyless invites crime, and where desperation and boredom lead people astray, as the following extracts make clear:

I do believe unemployment is the root cause of the growth of crime. It's not the cause of crime because there'll always be crime, and I just see that, you know, the kids that are about are not evil by nature but just through boredom and despair commit crimes.

There's the usual vandalism and this sort of thing. I feel sorry for them. What is there for them to do?

I think it is because you have a great melting pot of all layers of society, and in this area, which I consider a predominantly middle-class, yuppy-type area, you've got on the doorstep places which are socially deprived, and I think where you've got areas coming together like that, you are going to have problems. I think crime is rooted in those sorts of problems – social deprivation, unemployment, the fact that our society is becoming extremely divided. We've got a group of people who are just being squashed, really. So a step in the right direction, in levelling out the crime rate, would be to level out the division in society.

Responsibility for crime is thus diffused, with attention diverted away from the offender and associated negative images and stereotypes. Concern about crime is mediated by understandings and 'knowledge' of the causes of crime, many of which are seen as problems in their own right. Fear of crime and indeed understandings of what *is* crime is a narrow concept in the public eye, and it is an error to conflate crime with all life's irritations and life's problems.

## CRIME CONCERN, OFFICIAL REPRESENTATIONS AND THE MEDIA

An important question relating to fear of crime concerns the influence of the media in shaping people's views. It is well established, for example, that stories of violent crime in general and of sexual offences in particular are over-represented in the media (Gordon and Heath, 1981; Ditton and Duffy, 1983; Minogue, 1990) and it might be thought that there would be a strong likelihood that people's views of crime would be distorted by such accounts, since people in a neighbourhood 'may not have good individual knowledge of their collective experiences' (Skogan, 1986, p. 210). A constant diet of sensationalized accounts, concentrated upon atypical offences, might thus be expected to lead some people into unjustified concern about their own chances of being victimized (cf. Grade, 1989). Research, however, suggests that while exposure to such press coverage increases general concern with crime as a social issue, there is no consistent evidence that reading about crime is associated with higher levels of fear (Tyler, 1980; Skogan and Maxfield, 1981). The ability of the media to increase concern about crime as a social problem without also influencing personal concern of crime is thought by some writers to be linked to the 'illusion of vulnerability': even though aware of crime in the abstract, individuals may think that personal danger is unreal until they have been themselves victimized (Tyler, 1980, pp. 32–3).

Our research helps fill out these findings. In undirected questions, people very often mentioned the newspapers as sources of information about crime in the area. This is entirely understandable since research shows that learning from others and their experiences is important and rational for events which are rare but of high consequence when they occur (McIntyre, 1967; Skogan, 1977; Tyler, 1984). Residents also reported that they were aware of the possible influence of the press:

> I would not go out at night without a car. Now ten years ago, that would not have been the case. If I just walk down to the shops in the dark, I would take the dog.
>
> I think a lot of that is brought about not by policing but by the media, because all the time they're telling you how vulnerable you are, how many muggings there have been, and whilst there are a lot of these instances, if you look back to Victorian times there were at least as many rapes then as there are today. But today you have it thrown down you.
>
> It is wrong that I, at five foot eight inches, active, reasonably forceful, should be nervous about walking from here on my own at night.
>
> Now, that said, a quarter of a century ago a friend of mine had her handbag snatched in —— Road, so, you see how much I am influenced by what I hear on the radio, and by people's complaints.

Whilst conscious of the influence of the media, in general people were not willing to accord media accounts much weight in terms of the likely impact of crime upon their own lives until they had some empirical confirmation of the stories:

*Inner-city resident*
Q: Do you think that crime is a serious problem in this area?
A: You can only relate to what you've encountered. I've heard stories: the first impression you get round here is it's near St Paul's, the riots, muggings, beatings up, but I haven't come across these things.

*Suburban resident*

Q: Is there a crime problem in this area?

A: Not that I know of. I don't really know.

Q: What do you think?

A: Well, I haven't heard of much crime. I read about it, but I haven't really seen any or experienced any at all.

*Suburban resident*

Q: Is there a crime problem in this area?

A: I hear so much of it, read the *Gazette* every week but it is not really real to me because I don't see any of it.

But if the media influence is weak at the personal level, there is evidence that it is stronger at the abstract level (Tyler, 1984) influencing, for example, judgements about the rate of crime (Doob and MacDonald, 1979) and the demographic characteristics of victims and offenders (ibid.). Our study strengthens these conclusions in one important respect: official and media representations of crime have helped create and confirm a view that crime is predominantly committed by black people.

## Racism and crime

The way in which a 'moral panic' about the involvement of black people in crime was created by the police (whose bias against socially disadvantaged and powerless sections of the community is demonstrated in Young, 1971 and Box, 1981), judiciary and media has been well documented in relation to the 'mugging' scare of 1972–3 (Hall *et al.*, 1978). More recently, in 1982 and 1983 the Metropolitan Police issued statistics broken down by race, which purported to demonstrate over-representation of black people in crime. Despite basic flaws in these statistics (on which see, Blom-Cooper and Drabble, 1982; Kettle, 1983; Harris, 1983) media coverage was such as to justify Peirce's conclusion that 'the simplistic equation "Black = Crime" has been firmly established' (Peirce, 1982). What is apparent from our research is that, irrespective of the fact that the rate of involvement in crime by black people is unknown, the effects of such stereotyping can be far longer lived than the concept of 'moral panic' implies. Thus, years after the intense press coverage of the early 1970s and early 1980s, a few people spontaneously told us that crime was essentially a black problem, a 'fact' which had been officially established. Thus:

The coloured bloke over the road was arrested, carted away, but there was never any report in the local rag about courts or anything. That makes me suspicious of the reverseful workings of discrimination. The reverse to racial discrimination . . . in other words, it's positive discrimination inasmuch as because they're coloured they [the police] do bugger all about it because if they do they scream racial discrimination.

And I don't know whether you get to grips with any of this stuff down here in London, but a few years ago the Chief Constable of London was saying he'd had x amount of crimes, and actually on those crimes categorised who did what, where and when. The hammer came down in favour of the coloured majority – for petty crime, mugging, breaking and entering, drugs and the like. It came down in their favour. There's good and bad in all races, but there is an overwhelming majority on these figures, and they screamed murder about it.

What I've heard on TV and read in the papers, the majority of crimes are done by coloured people. I'm not saying they're all bad but they don't want to seem to communicate with the police because they say the police are picking on me.

I'm suspicious of groups of West Indian guys really, aged 15–20. . . . It's a terrible thing to say, I know, and if a West Indian person heard me say it I'd think they'd be raging, but at the same time I think somewhere in the more responsible sections of their community they recognise in their hearts that the small minority amongst them cause the rest of them a lot of grief. I mean, it's statistically proved in London that the worst violent crime is committed by West Indian people.

It is clear from this that negative representations of black people, 'legitimated' by officially-generated statistics, have fed directly into people's understanding of crime patterns. And it is therefore not surprising that these sentiments are carried over into the concerns of residents – which people they regard as suspicious, which people give them feelings of apprehension, who causes them concern and fear. As we shall see in more detail in Chapter 4, people frequently reported that they were concerned about black people either individually or in groups and this was also true of areas which were entirely white and of rural areas which had no contact with black people:

*Suburban resident*
Suspicion? This may sound very racist, but it would have to be someone who's black, simply because there aren't any here.

*Suburban resident*
If I saw someone coloured or looking in a funny way at my house, or at the other houses, I would think 'what's he doing here?' because we know all the people who go up and down the road. So, it's not a very nice thing to say, but that's that.

*Village resident*
Probably around here, because I don't think there's many coloured people, then probably a coloured person.

*Suburban resident*
Suspicion is something you feel at the time, something you can't explain – people standing anywhere, just looking, I don't know really. I get a bit wary now when there's more than a couple of coloured people walking towards me or behind me. My hand grips tight round my purse.

*Suburban resident*
There is burglary, house-breaking [in this area]. So far as I'm aware, there's no violence, or anything like that. There is the occasional mugging, but it's not really prevalent, really because I think anybody who is seen in that sort of stereotyped category as a potential villain – and that would have to be a young black person – would really raise the suspicions of a lot of people, to see a black youth, or maybe two black youths just cruising up and down the road at 11.00 o'clock at night, because this [area] is becoming increasingly a middle-class bastion which is exclusive of black people, even though there are black people in the road. Do you get the drift of it?

This is simply one graphic illustration of the way in which the 'crime problem' is socially constructed by the police and other state officials in ways which advance the argument of those who seek increased police powers and a 'stronger' state (see also King, 1989).

## CONCLUSION

Awareness of and concern about crime is widespread in Britain today. At its highest, it can effect profound changes in people's lives casting a deep shadow over everything they do, restricting their 'public' activities and turning each day into a lived nightmare. However unrelated to actuarial risks of victimization, fear of this kind must not be underplayed in any analysis. There is substance in the argument of the new realist criminologists that fear of crime cannot simply be a matter of statistical probabilities but is instead an intensely subjective experience. The evidence suggests that fear of crime is most intensely felt by women, a greater proportion of whom report concern about crime; and men themselves are identified as one of the central problems for women. Fear of crime also runs into general beliefs about crime and it is here that official and media negative representations of black people have disturbing effects. The successful linking by the police and the media of black people to crime increases and focuses fear of crime in areas of heterogenous populations and is also a feature of white suburban and rural areas. If not yet at the levels found in the United States (where 'white urban flight' characterizes many major cities, Farley et al., 1978; Skogan, 1986), concern about 'strangers' and 'outsiders', suspicion of people who 'do not fit' and who 'do not belong', and categorization of people as being 'good neighbours', is in England and Wales becoming a coded way of talking about black people. Fear of crime is, therefore, in a variety of ways a matter of personal, political and sociological significance to which we shall return later in this book.

None the less, we cannot agree that fear of crime should occupy a central position in thinking about law and order issues. Our research suggests instead that in the ordering of people's priorities, crime is of subordinate status, and, insofar as it constitutes a problem, is characterized by concern and not fear. In all our lives, concern about crime has some reality – we are taught to keep things safe, to lock things up, to avoid talking to strangers, and to keep away from certain areas. These become ways of thinking about our lives which are embedded in how we fashion our behaviour, in our regularities and routines. For most people, thinking about crime never becomes more than this and in their daily lives, as we have seen, problems other than crime have more resonance for citizens. The new realists' association of crime with war, 'where clear malice is intended' and, as in the following passage, with other forms of social disorder, do not reflect life's realities:

Crime is the end-point of a continuum of disorder. It is not separate from other forms of aggravation and disorder. It is the run-down council estate where music blares out of windows early in the morning; it is the graffiti on the walls; it is aggression in the shops; it is bins that are never emptied; oil stains across the streets; it is kids that show no respect; it is large trucks racing through your roads; it is streets you do not dare walk down at night; it is always being careful; it is a symbol of a world falling apart. It is lack of respect for humanity and for fundamental human decency.

(Lea and Young, 1984, p. 55)

Our research demonstrates clearly that people do *not* conflate social ills in this way; they do not have an apocalyptic view of social disorder and they carefully discriminate between activities which they are prepared to label crime, activities which deserve disapprobation but not utter condemnation, activities which are understandable even if not condoned, activities which are to be viewed indulgently because they are produced by some wider force, and activities which, though technically illegal, do not warrant criminalization. And overall, in the hierarchy of life's concerns, crime is generally subordinate to the destructive effects of bad housing, poor schools, unemployment and other social evils.

# Chapter 4

# The reality of neighbourhood watch

Crime and the fear of crime have been presented as increasingly serious social problems, their prevention or containment continually forced high on the political agenda. The 'crime problem' constitutes a standing demand that politicians do something to combat threats to order and to create in people a well-founded sense of security. In the most recent past, however, there has been a conscious attempt to delegate responsibility for crime, to make dealing with crime a civic duty rather than simply a matter that can be laid at the door of the police. In this initiative, neighbourhood watch is put forward as one of the central vehicles through which collective community action may be co-ordinated and expressed by 'active' citizens.

This conception of neighbourhood watch has to be seen against the background of an important debate between two conflicting sociological models of the relationship between crime, fear of crime and people's responses to these (see Skogan, 1981). On one view, crime is essentially something which fractures communities, eroding their capacity to exercise informal social control. According to this model, advanced by Conklin (1975), crime and fear of crime generates insecurity, suspicion and withdrawal from community affairs. Residents develop a negative view of their own localities, neighbourly interaction diminishes, with the result that the community is even less capable of exercising informal control. Although, as Skogan (1981, p. 73) points out, recent evidence tends to favour this explanatory model, it is the other one that has attracted political support.

The earlier model was that advanced by the French sociologist, Emile Durkheim (1933). In Durkheim's view, crime has an essentially integrative function. By shocking the sentiments of ordinary people crime stimulates them to act individually and collectively: community solidarity and morale are thereby increased, and informal social control exercised by the collectivity is strengthened. In the United States of America, this kind of thinking has been taken up by advocates of the 'social control' model, who see crime and fear of crime as indicators of the erosion of informal social control processes that are believed to establish and maintain order in society (Wilson, 1975; Wilson and Kelling, 1982; Kelling, 1986). The central argument is that 'collective neighbourhood efforts can influence crime and fear of crime . . . community crime control works' (Kelling, 1986, p. 91).

This social control model has been highly influential on official thinking about crime issues and is central to official conceptions of NW. Even if NW does not have a marked influence upon rates of crime or if its effects are hard to measure, the expectation is that NW will help deal with the problem of fear of crime:

> Implicit in NW is that fear of crime will be alleviated as residents come to have more of a sense of control over crime, both through their own efforts and those made on their behalf by neighbours.
>
> (Mayhew *et al.*, 1989, p. 59)

Irrespective of whether NW reduces crime, therefore, the theory is that it will act as a catalyst in bringing people together and re-creating a lost sense of community (Du Bow and Emmons, 1981).

In this chapter we shall explore the extent to which NW is successful in meeting these aspirations. We shall do this by examining, in the areas in which it has been established, whether it has managed to attract and maintain public interest and commitment to it; whether it has changed the behaviour of members in terms, for example, of crime security and crime surveillance; and whether it has brought people together and created feelings of solidarity. We shall also look at areas which do not have NW schemes in an attempt to understand why NW has not been established in these areas, whether residents would be in favour of schemes being established locally, and whether residents' behaviour in terms of crime and crime prevention is qualitatively different from those in NW areas.

## NEIGHBOURHOOD WATCH SITES

### How many residents are members of NW?

In two recent national British surveys, approximately one in seven respondents reported that they were members of NW (Mayhew *et al.*, 1989; Crawford *et al.*, 1990), a proportion double the membership rate in the United States (Whitaker, 1986) but only half that of Canada (Nuttall, 1988). Our findings demonstrate that, apart from differences between NW and non-NW areas, there are striking differences in the proportion of people who claim to be members *within* designated NW sites. Because we had difficulties in locating NW in other socio-economic groupings, our sites reflect the predominantly middle-class, white, home-owning bias that research shows characterizes membership of NW in general both in Britain (Donnison *et al.*, 1986; Crawford *et al.*, 1990) and the United States of America (Greenberg *et al.*, 1985; Skogan, 1987). As a result of this we could not test adequately whether membership in our sites varied in terms of type of accommodation, although it seems fairly well established that membership is greater among owner-occupiers than residents in other types of housing, both in Britain and the United States of America (Crawford *et al.*, 1990, Table 3.27; Garofalo and McLeod, 1989, p. 330). We found no factor which was able to explain the variations in membership that occurred across our sites and set out in Table 4.1.

*Table 4.1* Membership of neighbourhood watch as reported by residents

| NW site | Members, % | Non-members, % |
|---------|------------|----------------|
| 1       | 33         | 67             |
| 2       | 20         | 80             |
| 3       | 100        | 0              |
| 4       | 67         | 33             |
| 5       | 67         | 33             |
| 6       | 62         | 38             |
| 7       | 17         | 50             |
| 8       | 50         | 50             |
| 9       | 50         | 33             |
| 10      | 90         | 10             |
| 11      | 17         | 83             |
| 12      | 78         | 22             |

*Note:* In sites 7 and 9 a number of respondents answered 'don't know' when asked whether they were members of NW, and for that reason the percentages do not add up to 100.

People were attracted to join schemes for a variety of reasons. The positive image that NW has enjoyed and the prospect it offers for the reduction of crime and increase in collective security, were primary motivating factors, as the following quotations illustrate:

> [We joined] mainly because we've had experience of burglary and I hate these people who rob ordinary people. I take a strong moral view. People felt more secure and happy in their homes during [World War II]; but with prosperity it seems dreadful that people don't feel safe and secure in their own homes.

> It's for our benefit overall. It certainly helps keep crime down.

Sentiments of these kinds were sometimes linked to the view that the fight against crime imposed a civic responsibility upon everybody and that it was unreasonable to expect the police to deal with the problem on their own. In a few cases, however, residents expressed misgivings about what they saw as the transfer of responsibilities from the police to the public.

> It's in everyone's interests [to join] and the police aren't going to be able to do everything. I mean, the more people you've got caring about what goes on in the community, the less child abuse, the less old ladies molested, the less old ladies and old gentlemen falling downstairs and not being seen for three days, and so on.

> [We joined] to protect our little area I suppose because you don't get enough protection from the police, because they're not about. Even though I think its a way of them off-loading their responsibilities, you've got to look after yourself and your neighbours.

There was a sense among some residents that, whatever their personal feelings about the value of NW, they should join in order to show neighbourly solidarity ('Basically, I joined because everybody else was going in, so I went along with them'; 'I joined because of neighbourliness'). Perhaps surprisingly, only a few people mentioned instrumental benefits as reasons for joining: the offer of a free home security survey by a police crime prevention officer, the availability of property marking and, in some areas, a reduction in house insurance for members of schemes. And many residents reported that they had no clear reasons for joining and had not given the matter much thought but had agreed to join when requested to do so by a friend or neighbour.

In general, there were three things which led to people not being members: (i) some were not aware of the scheme; (ii) a larger group were opposed to the idea of NW; and (iii) the most numerous group could not be bothered to join. We shall say a little about each in turn.

### Unaware of NW

Although all our NW schemes had been commenced with an official launch meeting to which all residents were invited, and although each was signposted as an official scheme area, some local residents did not appreciate that there was a scheme covering their road or block. Some might understandably overlook an invitation to the official launch where the existence of a scheme might be expected to be most dramatically represented, and others might not notice NW signs in an area that is already so familiar to them that it does not require constant examination; none the less ignorance of the scheme is also indicative of a serious lack of impact by NW on the community. Whatever the precise reasons, some residents in NW sites asserted that 'there isn't any as far as I know in this road', or less dogmatically 'I think there is, or there was a neighbourhood watch scheme going on around the area. There is at the top; I'm not sure whether this road is involved', or more surprisingly:

Q: Are you aware of a NW scheme in this area?

A: I don't know whether there is one officially, in this immediate area, I think if I was to notice that there was somebody suspicious, something very strange going on anywhere, I'd do something about it. I'm sure there is a NW, but I don't know whether there is for sure; without me knowing for sure, I'd do something about it, anyway me personally.

Q: There is actually a NW scheme in this area. In fact you live next door to both of the people who are involved as co-ordinators. Have you not noticed the stickers in people's windows?

A: No.

Q: Would it actually make any difference to the way you saw things if you knew this place was a NW? Would you feel more secure?

A: Not really no, because the actual community, the people here, I feel secure in myself in as much as I didn't realise there was a NW scheme, and yet, I knew and felt that we'd all look out for each other anyway.

### Opposed to NW

A more substantial number of residents had not joined NW because they were actively opposed to the idea of it or were sceptical as to the motives of 'activists' or of the police. The most commonly given reason was that NW would not be restricted to activities which involved helping each other out but would spill over into 'snooping'. This illustrates the very fine line between good neighbouring and bad neighbouring, the latter including overstepping perceived boundaries of privacy (Bulmer, 1986, p. 33). Thus:

It's good that neighbours should be encouraged to take some responsibility, but there's always somebody who goes overboard and starts snooping.

No I am not a member, but I am sure they must have a scheme because they are awfully nosey. . . . I think old people have nothing better to do with their time than to look out of the window and watch what people are doing. I think old people want to see things that aren't there for one. I mean there could be a perfectly good reason for why someone is doing something but because they are out there looking for a criminal, or looking for someone doing something wrong, even if there is a logical reason for someone doing what they are doing, they will look at it in a different way.

You [can] get people who are too keen, they take the law into their own hands; go over the top, looking for every little thing. Cause more harm than good. Any sort of scheme like that is going to encourage the 'loony' element I suppose.

Comments of this character reflect concerns which have been advanced by critics of officially sponsored crime initiatives in general (Cohen, 1979; Mathieson, 1980) and of NW schemes in particular (Donnison et al., 1986; Gordon, 1987) that they might lead to greater control of the community, extending the reach of the criminal justice system:

I'm slightly suspicious of those [NW] schemes because, the whole idea of community policing, I'm not over-keen on what the police do and I'm not that keen. I think it can turn into a snoop system and I'm not sure that I want to be involved in that.

For other people, NW was seen as socially divisive, orientated around property and essentially a middle-class project:

I dislike the ideology that it is formed within, you know, about private ownership and that. There is something very middle-class about it, the way it started in the Tory shires. No, I don't feel particularly happy with it.

I don't want to use the word 'yuppy', but there are quite a lot of professional middle-class people moving in round here and spending a lot of money and are prime candidates for burglaries. They will be the kind of people who join a NW.... I think the whole idea that some houses have stickers in them and some don't, I think it's divisive. If I see a sticker in the window, it does give me a feeling of 'I've got something worth nicking and you haven't', sort of thing. Bit like burglar alarms really. It's a status thing really. . . . I don't know if the people who do neighbourhood watch know the police. Anyone who knows the police is going to get different or kid gloves type treatment . . . I mean my parents actually live quite close to here, and I don't think they are part of a NW scheme. They could be, and I would find it hard if they were part of something and getting different kind of treatment from what I would get, depending on what the house looked like from the outside. It could be quite a divisive thing.

*Could not be bothered to join*

By far the largest group, however, were those who, for one reason or another, simply could not be bothered to join. If NW is to be judged by its ability to fire the enthusiasm of residents enough in the early stages to ensure that they see NW as something they should join and to which they should devote a small amount of social energy, for a significant minority in scheme areas, NW must be judged a failure. These people were ones who said that they would require a special invitation, who had not joined because they missed the launch meeting, or who, in their own terms, did not see it as important enough to make any effort to join. The following quotations illustrate these sorts of viewpoints of residents who were asked to explain why they were not members of a local NW scheme:

> No one has asked us or come to us. Probably partly our fault, partly theirs. If it was going, they would come round I suppose.
>
> I haven't been invited to join. If someone asked me and invited me along to a meeting I would go I think.
>
> Actually I'm not [a member] because on the two meetings that were held I was at work.
>
> Couldn't be bothered!
>
> I don't know quite honestly. Maybe something else was happening at the time, or I forgot all about it.

**What does 'membership' involve?**

Any attempt at measuring membership rates within NW immediately runs into the difficulty that 'membership' has no settled meaning. There is no official definition of what constitutes membership or of what membership entails. The official Home Office publication *Practical Ways to Crack Crime: The Handbook* (3rd edition, 1989), for example, talks both of NW covering households and of it covering individual residents, making it unclear whether schemes are property- or people-based. This ambiguity reflects an embedded contradiction in official representations of NW: whilst efforts have been made to refute the suggestion that NW is essentially an activity of middle-class property owners, recruitment is invariably based on households, and the indicia of membership (stickers and signs) designed for property.

The ambiguity is apparent in the way in which residents address the issue of NW membership. Some people claimed membership on the basis that the house was in the scheme, evidenced by stickers put up by another (multiple-occupancy) household member or by previous occupants. Others saw membership as entirely personal: 'I'm in it but my husband's not', 'I think my parents are', being typical responses in this category. Yet others claimed membership on the basis that they lived in a NW area, even though they had not been to any NW meetings, put up NW stickers, or participated in any of its activities. Here are some examples of the ways in which residents understood 'membership':

> I believe we are [members]. The previous occupant was and we get things through the door. I presume it carries on.

> Me personally, no; but I think this household is.

> Q: Are you a member of NW?
> A: I am, I believe.
> Q: Why did you join?
> A: I don't know if I did join. I bought this house about twelve months ago and was told that I was a member.

> We haven't gone to NW meetings but we had a NW sticker on the door which we haven't taken off and we get reports every now and then. . . . When we moved into the house we had a NW sticker on our door and we are deemed to be part of the NW community.

> I think we are members – I'll just ask. [Pause while resident speaks to partner] The answer is we haven't actually paid our subscription yet but we have said we will. To all intents and purposes, apart from actually paying for the subscription we are in it because we said we would join. That's probably why it has slipped our minds in the last couple of months.

> [This woman] came to the door. She didn't give you an option, it was very interesting. She said: 'I am starting a NW, and here is your information. If you have any questions, like 'phone numbers, I live at so and so. Bye!' That was it. I wasn't asked if I wanted to join – 'You *are* joining'. And I thought 'it was easy to join'!

> *Resident in non-NW area*
> Our local bobby gave me the NW stickers when we had our burglary in August, and he marked our property and all that. Then when the proper Crime Prevention Officer came I told him about the stickers and he said 'Well, no, I don't want you to have them unless you're in NW, because that then makes it difficult for us, y'see . . . not knowing'. I turned to our bobby; 'You told me to put them up'. So they argued, but I kept it up, and so has next door.

The membership figures set out in Table 4.1 above cannot be

regarded as anything other than 'soft'. People understood membership in different ways and having a sticker, put up personally or inherited, was seen by most as equivalent to having joined a scheme.

## What do members of NW actually do?

### Attendance at meetings

The ambiguity relating to the meaning of 'membership' has implications for the theoretical basis of NW. Emphasis on signs, stickers and households speaks to a theory of crime prevention based on 'target hardening' through the creation of psychological barriers which are intended to deter potential criminals. This approach does not necessarily require efforts on the part of residents beyond the erection of signs and the posting of stickers. Although this might be the understanding of some residents, the Home Office and the police have encouraged activities linked specifically to NW, such as looking out for suspicious activity, as well as using NW as a vehicle to promote other crime prevention activities, such as property marking. There is also a more general hope that NW will promote a sense of community and thereby strengthen informal networks of social control.

Research suggests that a launch meeting can be successful in creating or reinforcing awareness, disseminating information, and stimulating activity, at least for a short period (Garofalo and McLeod, 1988). Our research uncovered only a minority of people who said that they had attended a launch meeting. Of those who did, experiences were variable. On the negative side, what was on offer did not meet the, in some cases exaggerated, expectations of residents, as the two following illustrations show:

> My mother was very keen on NW . . . but she didn't really feel that the police came out with much at the end of the day. It was, you know, 'Put your sticker on your window and here's our number'. I think she wanted something a bit more constructive, like a direct line to Scotland Yard, or something . . . but I didn't feel that she felt any better about it. I think probably if they'd said something like 'well, there'll be somebody on a beat going past your house every two hours', or something *definite*. It's very kind of remote, a police station and a number for old people.

The police threatened us with 'Oh yeah, if the meetings aren't going, we'll come and take the signs away because it costs x amount of pounds to put it up'. Y'know, it's the 'you don't play football the way I want it, I'm taking my ball back', know what I mean? Disgusting, really. So, I never bothered going to meetings after that. That's the sort of attitude I don't like from the police.

On the positive side, some residents appreciated security advice that was given by the police, and where it was part of the 'package', information about the local policing system, including the name of the local beat officer(s). This was most marked in the Gwent rural site where the launch of NW was something of a local 'event' which, for a few residents, dramatized the fear of crime and provoked some instant response, as the following resident makes clear:

We had a public meeting in the village hall to get the thing going. . . . We told the [Crime Prevention Officer] we were interested in this NW and he came out with his staff and they showed us a video, gave us a good talk on the subject, and gave a lot of information regarding the possibilities for lower insurance policies etc. . . . Oh yes, they were very helpful. Some of [the residents] went crazy [about security] and overdid the thing of course. We've got one house that's like Fort Knox. His place, you can't approach the door without alarms going off. . . . He's spent £1,000 on his place.

The large majority of residents in all areas, however, did not attend a launch meeting. Moreover, although the third British Crime Survey (Mayhew *et al.*, 1989) found that 27 per cent of NW members claimed to have attended a meeting other than the launch meeting, in our research it is clear that whether they attended a launch meeting or not, residents do not generally attend further meetings if these are held. Our research is fully in line with American research which shows attendance at NW or Block Watch meetings at low levels (Schneider, 1986; Rosenbaum *et al.*, 1986; McPherson and Silloway, 1987). Almost everyone interviewed said that they had not attended meetings, or that meetings were not held, or that they did not know whether meetings took place.

*Surveillance*

NW is perhaps best known for the encouragement it gives to residents to engage in surveillance activity. People are urged to be the 'eyes and ears of the police', to look out for any suspicious activity and to contact the police in case of doubt. This conception of NW sets out to appeal to people's self-interest as well as to encourage a sense of partnership with the police in the fight against crime. Residents are encouraged to recognize the fact that the police cannot be everywhere at the same time and to share some of the burden of identifying potential offenders and deterring their activities. Whilst the police encourage individual surveillance they discourage 'vigilante' patrols.

Our research uncovered little evidence that surveillance activities of residents had increased as a result of NW. At its highest, it has created a greater degree of awareness in residents, as in the following example:

> Before NW, I wasn't actually keeping my eyes out then. It's actually made me more aware of what's going on.

In addition, it has, for some, lent a sense of legitimacy to their activities, converting 'nosey-parkerism' into acceptable social interventionism:

> It encourages you, not to be nosey, but to take an interest. Some schemes do take it too far, start poking their noses in. It's not that organized here; it's basically a bit nebulous but because it's there, you don't turn your back. If you're walking down the street and somebody gets mugged you don't cross over; you call the police. It gives you a licence to take an interest.

In most instances, however, if NW had any effect upon people's watching activities it was simply to confirm what they had already been doing. We found, as had Shapland and Vagg (1987), a substantial amount of low-level watching activity by residents on a highly localized basis, usually confined to a few houses each way down the street. Those who went round the neighbourhood at night walking a dog had a more substantial radius of watching but, in general, people occasionally looked out of the window or watched when something, such as a noise, attracted their attention.

> NW just sort of consolidated more or less what we already did but made it official. . . . Certainly, if I'm sitting in the front room

here, reading the paper, I'll be keeping an eye out. . . . If I'm driving round the local area and I saw anything untoward, I'd certainly report it.

. . . because he [resident's partner] does go out at night for walks and what have you, he couldn't do any more than what he was already doing in the first place. But if they want us to join the scheme, well, that's fine.

There was, however, no evidence of any organized watching activity resulting from NW or of any genuine uprating in the surveillance behaviour of individual residents in the research sites (cf. Garofalo and McLeod, 1988 for the USA position). Indeed, it became clear that there was no difference in the reported levels of surveillance activity between people who were members and those who were not members. Non-members in scheme areas were equally likely to claim to keep a look out; they simply reported that membership was not a prerequisite of being a good neighbour, as the following examples show:

I keep an eye on things as much as anybody. The fact that I'm not a member doesn't make any difference. The only difference is that I haven't got a sticker in the window.

The only thing I think about NW schemes personally is that I can't see the point in them, because if I saw somebody looking at my neighbour's house suspiciously, then I would be suspicious – I don't need the police to tell me that, so I don't actually think they're needed; it's better to be a good neighbour; they all seem to be like that anyway round here.

Q: Would you be more vigilant if you joined NW?
A: No, I would not. I am very watchful and suspicious. In fact, my wife sometimes laughs at me, some of the things I think of. I sometimes say: 'I think Mike is away', 'Well, how do you know?'; 'Well, he leaves his windows in certain positions, you see.' . . . I do as much probably as people in it: I'm alert without being nosey and poking into people's business.

### Household security

NW is used as a vehicle to promote better security measures in the home, a matter that is likely to be of some attraction to middle-class property owners. Nevertheless, previous research has shown that people are not particularly security conscious. Thus, Winchester and Jackson (1982) found, in a study of 450 households, that 95 per cent had either poor or partial security, and of those with good security, one in four respondents admitted to not locking up properly on the last occasion they had left their house empty during the day. This parallels findings relating to the security of people's motor vehicles (Clarke and Mayhew, 1980).

As we have already seen, NW has the potential for increasing people's security awareness, particularly through advice given at a launch or progress meeting, or through a follow-up visit to the homes of residents by crime prevention officers. Those who have been lax about securing their homes may be stimulated into action by targeted advice or by reassurance as to cost. Likewise, some will be deterred from taking the measures advised precisely because of cost (Bains, 1989). But security measures do not necessarily involve cost:

> The local crime prevention officer spoke at the meeting. It made you be extra careful when you answer the door. If you weren't expecting anyone you should have the chain on your door and you wouldn't open the door without a chain on.

This is not to imply that few people in NW areas employed some kind of security measures on their property. On the contrary, almost all people had some form of security, some of an elaborate nature, but in almost all instances this was already in place *before* the introduction of NW and was a product of people's general awareness, or because of prior victimization. Our research strengthens and reinforces the third British Crime Survey data which reported that about half of those who had a security survey or marked bicycles had done so before they became members (Mayhew *et al.*, 1989, p. 54). The following are typical of the responses of residents in respect of the influence of NW upon their household security:

> We haven't really done much different since NW. Sometimes we think that perhaps we should but we haven't got round to doing things like putting alarms in and this sort of thing. So we haven't really done more in the way of security.

> I've always taken the precaution of bolting doors, and not opening the front door to strangers, and seeing that every-

thing's locked up when I leave, and keeping an eye out for things. I was doing that before NW.

I don't think we've done anything that we could attribute directly to NW. What *has* spurred us on is being burgled twice in two years. That's why we have chained locks. We've always told neighbours when we've been going away and that sort of thing. But I don't think it's actually made that much difference to me.

*Community spirit*

One of the much-discussed problems in certain high crime or run-down inner-city areas is the lack of social solidarity or, at least, its reduced and intermittent nature. And one of the aspirations of NW is to foster social relations, to break down the barriers of suspicion and to create or rekindle feelings of community. In this way it is hoped to strengthen informal social control and reduce crime and incivilities.

On a conceptual level, there can be little doubt that bringing people together, as NW aspires to do, would assist in breaking down barriers of suspicion, help create feelings of solidarity at some level, and thereby reduce fear of crime insofar as it is based upon uncertain social relations. The success of NW in this respect is, however, reduced by its inability to attract people to meetings, so the opportunities for establishing relationships in this way are fitful. Where they do occur, however, NW can act as a vehicle for creating relationships and making people feel more at ease in their locality (Bennett, 1990).

I think we've got to know some people better. The people that back on to us have become close.

It's certainly brought a lot of people together that might not otherwise have talked to each other or met each other.

Interestingly, the biggest claim for success in this regard came from the rural site in Gwent. This small village, people told us, suffered from lack of communication between residents, which contributed to a feeling of loneliness and isolation. This was not linked to fear of crime issues but simply reflected the parochialism and individualism that can characterize country life. The introduction to NW brought people much closer together, according to residents:

> You can notice the difference, you can feel the difference. With this social club we're starting tonight, three of them are from NW and they hadn't even met; but now they come to the meeting, had a public meeting to get the thing going and we are starting this week. . . . As things are going, I'm quite happy about it; I think everyone is.

## Overall activity levels

Previous research suggests that NW engenders, at best, low levels of activity on the part of residents (Henig, 1984; Bennett, 1990). In line with this we found that 'activity' consisted in most cases in putting up NW stickers. The overwhelming majority of residents stated quite openly that they engaged in no activity beyond this and that their role was entirely passive (cf. Crawford *et al.*, 1990, who report a minority as being 'active' without saying what 'active' means). The following quotations illustrate this point:

> I went to the initial meeting, knew a certain amount about NW schemes, thought they were a good idea, collected a sticker which says 'your friendly neighbourhood policeman is . . .' and stuck it on the noticeboard inside my front door, and every now and then considered vaguely that I should inform my insurance company that I am a member of NW scheme and see whether they will reduce my house contents insurance. Apart from that I have not a great deal of involvement – I am not an active member of it at all.

> I stuck the thing in the window and that's it.

> Well, I'm a sleeping partner.

> What is my involvement with the scheme? Nothing really, passive.

Comments such as these demonstrate a more general point about NW, well attested in the American research literature, that even if the launch of a scheme is accompanied by a spurt of activity, most schemes fail or quickly become dormant, a point given little official recognition either by the police or the Home Office. People do not want to attend meetings at the expense of other social activities or engagements, they do not generally wish to assume responsibility for being a contact person (street or area co-ordinator), or get involved with the production of newsletters. After the initial launch meeting, 'meetings' are gatherings of area and street co-ordinators and do not generally involve other residents, who are simply not aware that such meetings take place. Newsletters in turn cease to come out regularly or at all, unless sponsored and produced by dedicated local police officers or by local businesses. Where they continue to be circulated, their contents make little impact upon residents but can serve to remind people of the need for vigilance in the midst of a local crime upsurge, or at periods such as Christmas when certain types of crime such as burglary may be common.

Whilst the third British Crime Survey data suggest that only 4 per cent of NW schemes can be classified as inactive, this inactive classification is based upon a scheme having failed to erect fixed NW signs, produce newsletters or leaflets, or keep members informed about the working of the scheme (Mayhew *et al.*, 1989, p. 55). Any more rigorous measure of activity would lead to the conclusion that the overwhelming number of schemes are dormant. Certainly in our research areas, which were mostly located in prime NW residential sites, no individual scheme could be said to be active except at the weakest level.

## NON-NEIGHBOURHOOD WATCH SITES

Because of the way in which our study was structured, we were not able to examine how NW is distributed across the country, but British Crime Survey data show marked regional differences in scheme coverage as well as a bias toward house-owning, above-average-income families in low burglary risk areas (Mayhew *et al.*, 1989). In our study, non-NW sites were selected so that they matched as closely as possible NW sites in terms of housing type and geographical location. We examined whether residents in these sites had considered starting up NW schemes, whether they were attracted to the idea of NW, and whether they felt that NW would make any difference if introduced into their locality.

### Had NW been tried?

It is a well-attested feature of NW schemes, as we have indicated, that, after an initial period of interest and activity, most groups become inactive or even dormant. It should, therefore, be no surprise that we found in many non-NW areas that the setting up of a scheme had been a topic of discussion in the community or had been suggested by some individuals without generating enough enthusiasm to get to a launch stage. In most cases, this is something that had been 'mentioned' by someone but not pursued, although in a few instances discussion was more formal or some approach had been made to the police but without immediate success. These various positions are illustrated in the following quotations:

> We were talking about having [NW] in this road but it didn't seem to get off the ground. The lady next door was going to find out about it, and then nothing happened after that. It was mentioned anyway and this was a few months ago, but we never discussed it again and I never thought to mention it because I was busy with my own work.

> Our local community centre was talking about it . . . but even the people on the committee said they wouldn't, even if they joined, actually display the sticker. Now I find that a bit strange. They seem to think it's more of a 'come-on' for a burglar, which I thought was a sad point.

> When I asked up at [the local police] station, I think they said there was going to be one here, someone had suggested the idea. But because of their queuing on the starting up of schemes, it wouldn't be for a year or so yet.

Overall, however, we did not encounter serious attempts to set up NW which had ended in failure. NW was something which formed part of social chit-chat, a topic raised and quickly discarded through lack of genuine interest and commitment.

## Would people like to have a scheme?

There is some evidence that NW is still a popular idea in the country as a whole. Mayhew *et al.* (1989) report that two-thirds of non-members questioned in the third British Crime Survey were willing to join a scheme if one were set up (p. 56), an outcome consistent with the finding of Husain (1988) that the most cited benefit expected from a scheme was 'a greater sense of security'.

Whilst our study provides general support for these findings, we found great variations in sentiment towards NW. We were unable to explain these variations in terms of the housing structure or demographic characteristics of residents. Our tentative conclusion is that variations arise because attachment to schemes and the idea of schemes is weak and the anticipated benefits (if any) few: people did not in general express deep enthusiasm for a scheme and there is a fine line between those who see it as beneficial or not harmful and those who see it as serving no useful purpose. Before illustrating how residents who were in favour of a scheme spoke about NW, we set out in Table 4.2 the overall proportions of residents who said they would like to see NW introduced into their locality.

*Table 4.2* Proportion of residents in non-NW areas who are in favour of the introduction of a scheme in their locality

| Non-NW site | In favour of NW, % |
| --- | --- |
| 1 | 83 |
| 2 | 67 |
| 3 | 28 |
| 4 | 50 |
| 5 | 60 |
| 6 | 22 |
| 7 | 10 |
| 8 | 50 |
| 9 | 86 |
| 10 | 37 |

*Note*: The highest attachment to NW was in areas 9 (rural Gwent) and 1 (suburban London), the lowest in area 7 (suburban London) and 6 (suburban Avon and Somerset). There was no obvious factor or set of factors which explained these variations in response.

Overall there was a broad understanding of the basic idea of NW among residents, who showed as deep a knowledge as those in NW areas. There were a few individuals who misunderstood aspects of the scheme (as, for example, thinking that NW involved organized citizen patrols) or of its associated benefits (one respondent, for example, thought that membership led to a reduction in local property taxes), but this was also true of areas which already have schemes.

*Those in favour of NW*

Those who were in favour of the introduction of NW and felt that it would bring positive benefits tended to speak in terms of collective security and social solidarity:

> It would be a good thing: we're all cut off now, everybody's drifting.

> I think to a certain extent it works. In as far as, whether it's statistically proven to work, people feel safer for it because they think that a sticker's like having a hungry alsation the other side of the door. They feel better for it and it makes them generally aware, makes them appreciate they've got a mutual interest.

Nevertheless, it has to be said that expressions of support for NW were generally lukewarm or coupled with reservations about its worth. Some people had no high expectations of any benefits it would bring, and others felt it would make little if any difference:

> It couldn't do any harm. I don't really feel the need of it because we've never had that great amount of crime here, but I don't think it would do any harm.

> It's a good concept, but you've got to have the community to do it.

> I'd like it round here because we could help each other to look after each other's property, life and limb. [But] for a lot of people here once five o'clock comes they won't go out, so they won't know who's on the streets. So NW might not be a viable thing round here.

*Those against NW*

Those who were not in favour of NW were clearer in their views and expressed them with more vigour. One group detected in NW a property bias which they opposed or felt inappropriate to certain areas. These individuals were quite clear that NW was essentially a middle-class idea which was not suitable for those in rented accommodation or for residents who, though house owners themselves, put people before property:

> In an area like [this urban site] where there are squatters which the council and private people don't want, it's in the interests of

the property holder to try to promote this idea. When you have a huge city with so many homeless, what's more important, keeping buildings empty or people getting a roof over their head?

It's *houses* don't forget that they are talking about, and it's basically for middle class or upper class areas. I can't really see NW breaking into the [adjacent] council estate.

A second group, predominantly but not exclusively in the inner-city areas, was not in favour of NW because of its association with the police. Most schemes historically have been police-initiated and those started by civilians are perceived to be (and usually are) based upon close liaison with the police. This linkage is, for some people, problematic, either because they have misgivings about police practices (discussed in more detail in Chapter 6) or because they feel that residents ought not to get involved with an activity that should be the sole responsibility of the police. These people were not persuaded of the desirability of a 'partnership' model of policing.

I would not give up any of my time for something the police get paid for.

To me it's the police's job. It's more to do with nosiness and interference as I see it. . . . I wouldn't be involved in it, I'll tell you that.

I would not be prepared to be involved because you are identifying yourself with the police and I don't want to identify myself particularly. I know they have got a job to do but I don't like their attitude and I don't like the way they go about things. And I don't care what they say, [in the police there is] racism; they are racist and always will be.

The other identifiable group, though small in number, were those who were in some way apprehensive about being publicly identified with NW. These residents were concerned that membership of NW or, in particular, informing on people who broke the law, would expose them to some form of retaliation:

If you report someone for pinching, the police are going to tell them who grassed and you're going to find out that in the next few months your house has been done over. There's no point in me being in NW.

> The police have got a pretty bad image and [NW] would put me at risk with people in this area because I know a lot of dodgy people. The way it goes at the moment, dodgy people have a good image and the police are pigs; and until they change that, it's not worth me dealing with the police.

For the rest, residents were against the idea of NW for a variety of reasons, including hostility to the idea of 'spying', a concern that it would promote a 'vigilante-type' philosophy, and a feeling that the whole thing is 'just a gimmick'.

## Would NW make any difference?

Because support for the idea of NW was so tepid in non-NW areas, it comes as no surprise to find that the overwhelming majority of residents felt that NW would make little difference to their area. At its highest, a few people felt that it might break down isolation and feelings of estrangement, and offer support and comfort to vulnerable sections of the community such as pensioners. In general, however, people, whether for or against the introduction of NW, felt that NW was redundant or would be ineffective. Those who saw it as redundant were people who claimed that their area already operated according to NW ideals:

> We've more or less got it here, if you know what I mean, because we watch out for each other anyway.

> There's probably a NW scheme without there being a NW scheme if you know what I mean; people keeping an eye out without you knowing.

> I think NW would be a good idea but personally myself we've been doing it for years. . . . We do it without thinking. We go next door and say 'We're going away next weekend, could you keep an eye on our house?' Or if we go away, we just take it for granted that they will keep an eye on the place.

The other group thought that NW would not make any difference either because it would not address the most important social (non-crime) problems, or because it would not repair severely-fractured social relations:

There's lots of other basic things that people need to have done on estates first, like making sure there's proper lighting, make sure that the flats people live in are decent first of all. It starts from there. A lot of people don't have any respect for where they live . . . because they live in such doss-holes.

I belonged to one in Camberwell and they did absolutely nothing. I don't believe in those staggering facts about stopping crimes at all. We all had stickers in the windows and signs in the street, we were the only house in the street that never got burgled. It wouldn't do any good round here. It might in nice, quiet, residential streets where every neighbour knows each other, it's much more a community; but here nobody is really bothered about the people around them.

It wouldn't do any good in all reality. You haven't got the spirit here to make the involvement worthwhile. I just think it'll dispirit people even more.

## IS NEIGHBOURHOOD WATCH A SUCCESS?

There are several ways in which the 'success' of NW can be judged. The first is purely subjective and is based upon whether NW is seen by residents as a useful mechanism which produces some social benefits. A second is whether NW is effective in reducing crime. A third is whether, irrespective of any actual impact on crime rates, it reduces fear of crime (this in turn would be 'success-ful' only to the extent that it reduced unfounded or irrational fear). Although we did not set out to measure directly the effects, if any, of NW on crime rates, our research provides useful information on each of these matters.

### Public perceptions of NW

In the official rhetoric, NW is a success story, with (according to official figures) an ever-increasing spread of schemes throughout the country. According to the latest national survey, about half of members thought that there had been benefits from the scheme, with over four in ten believing that NW had reduced crime (Mayhew *et al.*, 1989, p. 57).

In our study, only a very small minority (fewer than one in ten) of residents felt NW had been a success in their area. The few who judged it to be a success did so primarily on the basis of crime-related information contained in the local NW newsletter. Although this is obviously an insecure foundation for any evaluation, understandably a few people were influenced by such fragmentary material:

> It's definitely a success in this area. You've only got to see the monthly crime reports. In the June one, there were only two reports whereas before there used to be quite a lot.

> Reading the leaflets, it seems to be very much a success. There was no crime in April or May.

To a very limited extent, therefore, NW can become 'successful' if newsletters persuade people that schemes are successful or present crime figures in a manner which leads to this inference.

For the vast majority of people, however, NW was not deemed to be successful. In some cases, residents reached this conclusion precisely because they saw that reported crime had increased or because NW had not eliminated crime:

> The guy next door got his car nicked with his car alarm going off and nobody did a thing; so from that point of view it's not a success.

> NW I don't think has done any good at all because the crime rate's gone up in this road.

Ironically, the fact that NW has taken the firmest hold in areas which are relatively low-risk crime areas and has been marketed as an aid to crime reduction, has been instrumental in both its lack of impact and the negative evaluation given by residents. Sold as an anti-crime strategy, NW very often loses its rationale in crime-free areas, schemes quickly become dormant, and residents see the schemes as failures. Similarly, in communities which are virtually crime-free, NW can never be 'successful' if success is judged according to the ability to solve crime. This patterning, therefore, predictably produces negative assessments of the following kinds:

> I get the impression that the impetus has probably fizzled out.

> Its success depends on crime. As we haven't got any crime (as we were told by the police at the beginning) it will probably die, because there is nothing to keep it going.

I don't think there is the need for it here. . . . How can you achieve better than 100 per cent crime free, which is what we were before [NW]. I think it brought people together at the beginning, which has tended naturally to drift away a little bit.

Most residents went into NW without high expectations but recognized that they 'had nothing to lose'. Nevertheless, the lack of impact of NW left residents with the firm impression that NW was a non-event, aptly captured by one respondent in suburban London who said towards the end of our interview,

Why did you choose such a middle-class area for your survey? You should be in another area shouldn't you really? None of your questions are relevant to this road because nothing happens here.

Overall, when residents were asked specific questions about the effects, if any, of NW on their relationships with their neighbours, their relationships with the police, on community spirit in the locality, or on any other matter, responses confirmed the picture which is already clear: that, insofar as it was apparent to residents, NW had little or no discernible effects.

Those residents who were unsure whether it was successful or not withheld judgement on the basis that it was too early to make an assessment. Since, however, schemes had been in existence for a minimum of six months, and often for two or more years, these views must be regarded as further evidence of the failure of NW, since all the evidence points to activity levels being highest at and shortly after launch.

## Objective measures of success

Although we did not set out to measure directly the impact of NW, and share the view of Walker (1987) that a complete social science evaluation of NW programmes is not possible, we are none the less in a position to make confident statements about the worth of NW schemes in Britain today. Our conclusions add to a growing body of research which suggests that NW is ineffective in reducing or preventing crime, and has few other noteworthy benefits. Further, as will become clear below, our findings cast grave doubt upon the *potential* of NW as a crime-beating instrument even under 'optimum' conditions. There are three distinct points that come out of our research and require separate treatment.

### Subjective perceptions, objective effects

First, the subjective perceptions of residents (detailed above) have important objective consequences which cast substantial doubt on the value of NW. Residents who see NW as a failure or as unnecessary cease to undertake any collective activity (such as 'watching out') on which the model's theoretical value rests. Schemes become dormant, leaving their 'success' to depend upon the deterrent effects of the psychological barrier created by signs and stickers; and the evidence suggests that the decision-making of burglars is influenced by whether property appears to be occupied, rather than conventional target-hardening measures such as alarms (Reppetto, 1974; Walsh, 1980; Bennett and Wright, 1984). Even if stickers created some kind of psychological barrier, it is likely that their effects would be diluted as NW spread to adjacent areas: 'success' in terms of popularity is thus likely to reduce its worth. In any event, the overall inactive condition of NW reflected in residents' views is linked to two critical features encountered in the research: insofar as NW requires a base in fear of crime this is presently lacking in most areas of Britain, and, where it is present, NW is lacking. Further, and related to this, schemes quickly die because they did not emerge from the people themselves. Historically, they have not arisen out of a community demand but rather have been police-inspired. Given this, it is hardly surprising that most schemes have failed.

### Fear of crime

A second point to emerge from our research is that NW's strategy of seeking to exploit fear of crime runs the risk of *increasing* fear of crime. An increase in the fear of crime can lead to a further fracturing of social relations, thus weakening, not strengthening, community spirit and informal social control over crime and incivilities. As Iadicola put it,

> Instead of further integrating and interacting with other members of the community, residents may further isolate themselves and become increasingly suspicious of neighborhood activity.

The process of individually making their home and themselves more secure, may cut them off from others.

(1985, p. 144)

People do not generally possess grounded information about crime in their locality, and the stress upon security against *possible* crimes can create enhanced fear in individuals. This can also happen as a result of the provision of details of local policing, as the following interview reveals:

Q: How, if at all, has NW affected your relationship with the police?

A: It hasn't. It enabled me to see at first hand how ineffectual they were. I mean, it frightens me really, because I found out there were only eight policemen to cover the area at any one time.

Although there are indications elsewhere that NW might increase fear of crime (Rosenbaum, 1988; Bennett, 1990) its lack of penetration in the sites we studied showed no systemic effects of this kind. It remains, however, another embedded contradiction of the NW model.


*Divided outlook, divided response*

Central to the theory of NW is the assumption that people can be convinced of the desirability of surveillance activities and of the value of bringing to the attention of the police anything believed to be suspicious. We have already seen that this assumption is badly flawed insofar as it trusts in the capacity of NW to stimulate residents into understanding watch activities: for the most part, NW is wholly ineffective in this regard and the surveillance habits of members and non-members are indistinguishable. But this does not deal with a core issue: would residents contact the police if they saw something that was suspicious? The expectation of NW is that they would; evidence from previous research suggests that this is less true of certain groups in the community. It is to that research and its reasoning that we now turn.

An increase in the flow of information to the police from the public is seen as 'crucial to effective policing' by the new realist criminologists (Crawford *et al.*, 1990, p. 98; Lea and Young, 1984). Successful policing, in this analysis, requires a high level of public involvement in the criminal justice system, because most serious crime known to the police is reported to them by the public. An increase in the flow of information to the police would, on this argument, lead to more crimes being cleared up, which in turn would generate greater respect for the police and hence a further improvement in the flow of information (see the critique of this position by Ward, 1984). The crucial factor, therefore, is the willingness of members of the public 'to bring crimes to the attention of the police and participate in the judicial process' (Crawford *et al.*, 1990, p. 98). The surveys undertaken in Islington by the new realists suggest that a substantial number of people are unwilling to co-operate, particularly among women, the young, and black people.

Our research provides some support for their findings, as we shall see when we discuss public experiences of policing in Chapter 5. However, the Islington crime survey data were gathered exclusively from inner-city areas and it is not sensible to erect a general theory of public willingness to participate in policing activities on the basis of what may be atypical locations. To reach a fuller understanding, it is also necessary to incorporate into the analysis public attitudes in areas where confidence in the police is higher and where police–citizen relationships are positive. When this is done, a richer and more complex picture emerges, which has substantial implications for NW.

The first and basic point to make is that most residents have no real knowledge of crime in their area and very little crime-related information that would be of interest to the police. Very often people reported little understanding of crime matters and, even in high-risk areas, were ignorant of local crime patterns, which tend to be known, if at all, only to area and street co-ordinators, i.e. those who attend NW meetings. Indeed, some were distressed to discover from newspapers or general gossip that they lived in a 'crime area'. For most people the daylight hours are occupied with work, which oftens keeps them indoors or takes them outside their residential area. This means both that they cannot perform any surveillance function in their area during the day and also that the last thing they want to do at night is patrol the neighbourhood or look out of their windows. And in many areas, people are unable to look out for their neighbours because they live their lives in the 'back' of their houses and thus do not customarily scan the local streets for suspicious occurrences:

We joined because of neighbourliness. I thought if everyone kept an eye on things, well, it would be better wouldn't it. This neighbourhood watch business, we live in this [garden-facing living] room chiefly. We have a dining room in the front but, of course, we only go in there for meals, so we're seldom in the front of the house. So really we're not in a position to be very good at watching for most of the day.

Moreover, many suburban sites are distinguished by a high proportion of transient people (such as students, and people who switch accommodation addresses frequently) whose knowledge of and commitment to the area may be tenuous, as in the case of the following young London inner-city resident:

I don't really see that there are any problems because I don't want to get much out of the area: I live here and that's all I really want, so I don't use the area as much as I should. I suppose I don't know the area that well.

In the case of many people, therefore, it is pointless to ask them to pass on information, as they do not possess it. It would make sense only if they were encouraged to acquire such information, as by surveillance activity; but, as we have seen, NW is singularly unsuccessful in this regard.

A second point is that the NW model, and much of the discussion surrounding public–police partnership, rests upon questionable assumptions about people's *capacity* to respond to suspicious activity. It is assumed that if people witness a suspicious incident they can instantly contact the police, such as by telephoning. This may well be true of middle-class and other property owning areas, but it is much less true of poorer areas where people may be reliant upon public telephones. In the inner-city and council estates we found that this was something that figures prominently in people's decision-making:

Q: Would you call the police if you saw someone suspicious?
A: If I had a telephone I would, but the nearest [working] 'phone box from here is about two miles down the road.

Say I'm in [my flat]. I haven't got a 'phone, so it means I've got to run to somebody else to 'phone and that's something that I wouldn't do. If I see vandalism from here – one of them smashing one of these cars up – what have I got to do? Do I run to a 'phone, ring town [the main police station] or the local police and they farm it off to someone else. By the time it's finished up, the thing's done, finished, gone, and nobody knows.

A third point relates to the public's construction of suspicion. A failure to analyse how people understand suspicion has given rise to two misconceptions which underlie debates about NW. The police assume that residents understand suspicion in the same way as they do and will have a ready supply of low-level information to pass on to the police which easily slots in to existing police categorizations. Others, such as the new realists, have assumed that people can readily distinguish between criminal and non-criminal behaviour, and between criminal and non-criminal people. Neither of these assumptions accords with social reality.

The public have a much narrower conception of suspicion than the police and require much more evidence of wrongdoing before considering any social intervention. Reasonable suspicion for the police is anchored in well-documented stereotypes, and operates disproportionately against young, inner-city males, especially young black males. The young, unemployed and economically marginal are special targets. Suspicion is not simply stereotyping; it also founds and justifies police intervention, such as stop-searches and road blocks (Brogden, 1981; Tuck and Southgate, 1981; McConville, 1983; Willis, 1983; Southgate and Ekblom, 1986; Dixon et al., 1989). Public conceptions of suspiciousness sharply differ from those of the police.

In general, we found in our survey that members of the public were not willing to say that there was such a thing as a criminal type. In contrast to the police, therefore, the public were not generally willing to judge people on the basis of their hair-styles, dress or general appearance. Criminal typologies appear to be police- not public-based. When asked, 'What sort of person, if any, would arouse your suspicions in this area?', people generally refused to identify suspicion with categorizations of this kind, as the following examples show:

You can't really. There's no conformity is there? There's nothing that can be like criminals. Criminals are criminals, it doesn't matter what colour they are, what age they are. It could be a fifteen year old white youth or a twenty four year old black kid. Or it might be a watcher – a white woman – no one is going to notice her hanging around on the corner watching people going out from the flats, something like that. It could be anyone. You can't get a value judgement as to what a criminal is and what a criminal isn't. It's too easy to categorise, people always like to look for a scapegoat. Criminals are criminals and you don't know what a criminal looks like until you see him commit crime.

Nobody. . . . There's no uniform. You learn not to judge by appearances so nobody looks out of place.

This approach has a particular effect in the inner city and any other area distinguished by mixed populations. In the absence of crude stereotyping, people cannot identify, in heterogenous areas, individuals who are 'suspicious'; this was demonstrated to us time and again in the research:

Generally, you can't feel threatened because it's such a mixed community. . . . Round here there are so many possible types of people, you can't think to yourself 'they are odd' because they're *all* odd from one point of view!

NW is supposed to be a community that's helping to look out for suspicious characters I suppose and in that sense I'm surprised it's effective because I would have thought people either see nothing suspicious or see it on every street corner.

I believe that a lot of people look suspicious but that is just how they look. The rest of the people, there's a very wide cross-section of different types of people live round here, and therefore you wouldn't necessarily look suspicious because you were dressed in a particular way, or a particular age or colour or anything like that, since a wide variety of people live round these parts. I don't believe you ought to look at people and think 'Ho, ho, he looks suspicious because. . .' – you have got to be acting suspiciously.

Notwithstanding this, however, we encountered a very strong streak of racism in the attitudes of many people, especially in, but not confined to, city areas. For many, crime is associated with black people, and respondents were without prompting quite willing to identify ethnic minorities as the principal source of their crime concern. This was most striking in London, where some 36 per cent of white respondents in all areas spontaneously blamed black people for crime or made overt racist comments in the course of interviews with us. In the other police force areas, such comments were almost exclusively confined to the inner-city areas, with 31 per cent of Gwent and 25 per cent of Avon and Somerset inner-city residents making explicit racist comments. In addition, some respondents in all force areas, whilst not openly engaging in racist talk, spoke negatively about specific areas which have a high proportion of black residents, and others spoke in coded language about 'strangers' or 'outsiders', sometimes making it clear that this terminology was meant to include black people. Although, therefore, some respondents were diffident about exposing their prejudices to comparative strangers, a strong minority of residents in all force areas gave vent to their feelings. The following examples illustrate the sorts of attitude we encountered in this respect:

> Black people are dangerous animals. I shouldn't say this, but when [a mugging] happens, I hate all blacks. I don't normally allow a black in this house. . . . If you say to me who are the first football hooligans, I would say the British; they were the ones slung out of Europe. You say to a black that mugging is a black crime, crash! that's a red rag to a bull. They won't have it.

> They have got no manners and no respect. . . . They still think that they are living in a jungle and they forget themselves that they are living in England. . . . Half the white people have put their tail between their bloody legs and they've run, instead of staying put. Most of what the blacks do is mugging; they are 'steaming' and all that kind of stuff.

> If I was out and a black bloke came towards me, I'd be suspicious, and I'm not racialist at all, but if you are white you don't do that.

> I'm suspicious of dodgy people, especially black kids hanging around.

Even if people are suspicious of individuals because of their looks, colour, manner or dress they, unlike the police, appear unwilling to act upon the basis of their suspicion. What triggers responses in people generally is suspicious behaviour, and often behaviour which is unambiguously of a criminal character. This clearly emerged both in how people defined suspiciousness and in whether they would do anything on the basis of their suspicions, as the following quotations demonstrate:

> If I was suspicious, I would probably keep my eye on him, and if he actually does something that confirms my suspicions then I probably would call the police personally. I think I would hold back just to be sure.

> There's so many types of people about and they're all dressed differently. You can't go by dress, you can't go by looks, it would have to be vandalism or violence.

> Suspicion? A person who *acts* differently. You can't judge people by the way they look or walk. It doesn't matter if they are a punk or anything.

> I'm not a suspicious sort of person, really. I wouldn't say I'm actually gullible, but I don't really look out for suspicious events. A strange face might attract my attention. I might sort of wonder why and whatever, but . . . he'd have to definitely be doing something suspicious for me to regard them suspiciously. It would be more actions than appearance.

> I wouldn't be suspicious of any particular type of person, it would just be the general behavioural thing I think. . . . Unless I saw them doing something, I wouldn't do anything about it. I would have to see them doing something.

Encouraging people to inform more than they do presently therefore runs a severe risk that people will act not only upon behaviour thought to be criminal, but also upon categorizations of people thought to be suspicious. The effect of this would be to legitimate crude criminal typologies – the very thing, incidentally, which new realist criminologists themselves criticized in the 1960s and 1970s. It would also, of course, give a push to a further fracturing of social relationships and thus defeat one of the principal goals of NW. In most communities there is a balance that people strike, enabling them to live together, a balance which depends upon *not* knowing too much about neighbours (even if they are believed to be a bit 'dodgy') and *not* intervening unless the situation is clear. Whilst the police today, and historically (Pearson, 1989), believe that people who do not 'come forward' are deterred through fear of reprisals, residents are much more concerned to preserve their ordinary social relationships with others in the community. Acting precipitately, meddling officiously in situations which may be innocent, causes embarrassment, upset and even hostility of some kind, consequences which people are careful to guard against:

Q: Would you be tempted to call the police if you saw anything you thought was suspicious?

A: Not unless I was very sure of myself. I wouldn't want to get it wrong and upset somebody.

I don't think any person on their own would arouse my suspicions. Maybe if I saw a couple of blokes hanging about in a car, looking at a house, or a group of teenagers walking about, looking around. But, most of the things I've said, there's little point in 'phoning the police, because the person's done nothing wrong. In my opinion the police might think different: but if I was someone walking up and down a street and a copper came along I'd be quite annoyed, or if I was sitting in a car.

If I was suspicious, I'm afraid I wouldn't do anything. I don't like accusing innocent people.

Suspicionwise one tends to avoid things rather than be a Sherlock Holmes. You'd only create an incident if you barged into something that was quite innocent.

It's going to sound a bit two-faced because I said [earlier] that there was no neighbourhood spirit, but then again I don't get involved if it's nothing to do with me. Living here, sometimes you see and hear things that it is best not to see and hear: you could create trouble for yourself.

Of course, non-intervention in crimes like domestic violence operates at a different level of perception because

differential marital responsibility and authority give the husband the perceived right and the obligation to control his wife's behaviour and thus the means to justify beating her.
(Dobash and Dobash, 1979, p. 93)

In crimes of this sort women, as men's property in the home, are not only a focus for violence but are pushed into this position by the attitudes and ideologies in their wider communities.

## CONCLUSION

Crime is not a continuously salient issue in most people's lives. It is not for the most part central enough to drive communities together, as envisioned by Durkheim, or to drive them apart, as hypothesized by Conklin. Its association with fear of crime has not assisted the development of NW schemes, as American researchers have also found:

> There is substantial evidence that community organizations created solely to fight crime have neither long lives nor much success in recruiting members. Fear of crime per se is not much motivation for long-term collective action.
>
> (Taub *et al.*, 1984, p. 184)

Although some people are strongly opposed to NW, its failure to establish in most areas cannot be blamed upon organized community resistance. Rather, NW is not emergent and does not represent a genuine community demand. The launch of a scheme may bring benefits for some individuals, by teaching basic security principles and broadening their friendships within the neighbourhood, but the effects overall are insubstantial for NW as a social movement. Most schemes quickly become dormant, and those which may still be said to function at some level have a life only in the meeting of police and co-ordinators, and in the occasional newsletter. In broad terms, NW areas are indistinguishable from those which lack a scheme.

Our research agrees with other evaluations that NW cannot be described as a 'success' (cf. Husain and Bright, 1990). Members make no such claim and, apart from a few exceptions, are unable to point to beneficial structural changes relating to the reduction of crime and fear of crime, the improvement in home security systems, the creation of better social relations, or improved relations with the police. More rigorous measures of success demonstrate that the mechanisms designed to effect social change (such as increased surveillance) simply do not function. Moreover, any genuine attempt to operationalize these mechanisms runs the grave danger of stigmatizing and labelling significant sections of the community, further fracturing social relations.

# Chapter 5

# Police commitment to community policing

We have already seen substantial deviations from the official promises of neighbourhood watch. The picture of a successful, ever-expanding network of schemes moving towards comprehensive nation-wide coverage is far removed from the stark realities, documented in Chapter 4, involving low take-up rates, weak community penetration and limping, dormant or stillborn schemes. Moreover, the promise to provide community-based officers to answer the universal public demand for locally based, foot patrol officers, detailed in Chapter 2, has clearly not been met.

In this chapter, we begin to explore the extent to which the failure to deliver these promises is attributable to the ways in which individual forces have responded to the neighbourhood watch ideal. In the first section, we examine how the forces have responded at an institutional level in terms of sponsoring NW schemes, switching resources to community beat officers (CBOs), establishing selection procedures to identify officers particularly suited to community-based work, and instituting training programmes for them. In the second section, we look at the kinds of officer willing to engage in CBO work, their status within the force and their general morale. In the third section, we examine how CBOs carry out their tasks on a daily basis, the emphasis they give to neighbourhood watch, and the success they have in establishing and maintaining schemes. Finally, we examine the ways in which the police measure the value of NW schemes and the extent to which they consider them to be a successful innovation.

## THE INSTITUTIONAL RESPONSE OF FORCES

The three forces in our study are all officially strongly committed to community policing principles. Whilst 'community policing' is an open textured term 'often loosely used to accommodate virtually any policing activity which its proponents approve' (Weatheritt, 1987, p. 7), each force espouses a service model of policing, in which community consultation, the sensitive use of discretion, discussion, conciliation and negotiation dominate. Although no officer put forward a thoroughgoing model of the kind advocated by Alderson (1979), all senior officers to whom we spoke who had responsibility for NW schemes or 'community involvement' defined their job in community policing terms, and saw this as the way forward for the police. There was, for example, a strong emphasis upon officers dedicated to particular beats, who would get to know the community, and an acceptance of a shift in the balance that this implies (except in rural areas) from car to foot patrols. Alongside this, police policy-makers stressed the importance of officers establishing relationships with the community without the pressure to make arrests associated with 'fire-brigade' policing (a term used to describe a style of policing based upon fast response to incidents using patrol cars so that contact with the public only arises when the police are called upon to deal with a situation). Prevention of crime was seen as having greater value than apprehension of criminals. Neighbourhood watch was spoken of positively as a useful mechanism for both delivering and symbolizing the commitment to the needs and wishes of the community. There is, however, a gulf between the aspirations of these officers and the operational realities on the ground, which we shall now examine.

**Back to the beat?**

Since the late 1970s police forces throughout England and Wales have publicly embraced policies designed to 'return bobbies to the beat'. This has been an underlying theme of the moves towards bureaucratic rationalization, of the process of 'civilianization' of various tasks traditionally performed only by police officers, as well as of the implementation of community policing ideals. It has also been a feature of government funding policies. Thus, of the 430 extra posts approved in the provinces in 1986/87, 300 were placed in patrol and resident beat duties in specific areas (*Guardian*, 12 April 1988). To date, the objective of returning has been proved difficult to achieve, as earlier research establishes.

The study of the Metropolitan Police carried out in the early 1980s by the Policy Studies Institute (1983) found that only 6 per cent of constables were community beat officers. Although the proportions are higher in some provincial forces, radical changes there have been hard to effect. In Hampshire, for example, the Chief Constable reorganized the force in the early 1980s in order to bring about a definite shift of staffing from the uniform reliefs to the 'area beats' (Horton, 1989). Research by Smith and Horton (Smith, 1987), however, has shown that 'Even in Hampshire, where there has been a substantial transfer of manpower to permanent beats, they still account for only 15 per cent of officers up to the rank of inspector' (p. 59). Smith found the proportion of community beat officers in most forces to be typically about 5 per cent and concluded that outside Hampshire they were 'certainly not the bread and butter of policing; they are just a bit of icing on the cake' (ibid.).

Our study confirms these earlier findings. In all three force areas, community beat officers were a small proportion of all constables, being massively outweighed by uniformed relief officers. Uniform relief officers are organized into tight units, work together in shifts and are the first line of response when the public calls for police help. All the forces we examined were dominated by relief groups of this kind. Thus, in 1990, figures supplied to us by each force showed that community beat officers constituted approximately 7 per cent of constables in the Met. (1,400 out of 20,960), 13 per cent in Avon and Somerset (253 out of 1,959) and 18 per cent in Gwent (139 out of 755).

These figures reflect both an ambivalence in the commitment of forces to the beat officer ideal and a difficulty in matching demand to available resources. The ambivalence in commitment is displayed in the way in which community beat and neighbourhood watch structures are often poorly integrated into core policing work. In both the Metropolitan and Avon and Somerset Police, for example, officers were critical of the lack of co-ordination of various policing initiatives. Thus in London, senior officers in charge of NW in sub-divisions claimed to have little or no direction from the Crime Prevention Unit in Regency Street, as the following example shows:

> If you asked me what contact I have I would say 'as much as I want'. But if you say to me how often am I in contact with the

people at Regency Street, I would say 'very infrequently'. And if you ask me what do the people at Regency Street do in relation to neighbourhood watch, I would say 'I don't know'.

Officers involved in or in charge of neighbourhood watch routinely said that they had no contact with community involvement offices, community beat officers were, in Avon and Somerset and the Metropolitan Police District, often poorly integrated with relief officers, and in some areas of London CBOs said that they had no connections with the 'neighbourhood watch office'!

Historically, there has been a clear division between forces in the way they have addressed the question of the delivery of community policing. Both the Met. and Avon and Somerset embraced NW as an important delivery system in the early 1980s, and both saw value in NW being police-led. In effect, this meant that both forces took primary responsibility for NW, promoting and advertising its virtues and its availability, marketing it directly and through the media, and supporting initiatives through the production of newsletters. By October 1990, official figures showed over 1,770 schemes in Avon and Somerset (increasing at 30 to 40 per month), and some 10,160 schemes in the Metropolitan Police District (increasing at some 50 per month). The resource implications were not properly foreseen (Husain, 1990) and both forces have since the mid-1980s made substantial changes to this policy. Instead of the police selling NW, the emphasis now is upon citizen-initiated schemes supported by the police. Although the police still produce most of the newsletters, in each force schemes are encouraged to look for private sponsorship from the local business community and, in a few cases, this has resulted in a transfer of responsibilities from the police to private individuals. The consequences of this overall policy change will inevitably be a slow-down in the growth of new schemes and an acceleration in the demise of existing schemes. Thus community beat officers reported that the switch to private sponsors in their areas had attracted criticism from members of the public, who interpreted the change as a withdrawal of police support.

Gwent by contrast has never actively promoted the idea of NW. Its official policy is that NW can be helpful to both communities and the police, but that this is most likely to be so where schemes are truly emergent. In pursuance of this view, the force looks to residents to initiate schemes, guaranteeing police support if there is sufficient backing for a scheme from within the community. However, little publicity is given to this policy and it is a source of confusion among officers at both junior and senior levels. Indeed, most officers to whom we spoke understood the policy to be directed towards discouraging NW, as the following examples show:

*Gwent relief officer*
Nothing will change in the police, especially on a thing like this neighbourhood watch. If the Chief Constable has got an attitude towards it, which he does on this force, then his attitude goes, because he is the boss. If he doesn't want it here, then he won't have it here.

*Gwent community beat officer*
The Chief Constable is dead against NW. Absolutely. He thinks it is bad, because he doesn't think it is the way to police, to get people to spy on each other. He thinks you end up with vigilante groups on the estates and things like that. I disagree with him, but that's his reasoning.

The predictable result was that by the middle of 1990 there were only eighteen schemes in the whole of Gwent. Residents rarely attempted to initiate schemes and, where they did, officers could give them little encouragement. Indeed, in a number of cases officers told us that they were unsure how to deal with enquiries of this sort.

## Police training

The gap between the official rhetoric of the forces and ground-level realities is, however, most clearly displayed in the areas of staff deployment and training. The theory of community policing is that a CBO will be dedicated to a particular beat and in that way gain knowledge of and acceptance by the local residents. Research carried out by the Home Office in the early 1980s found, however, that community officers were frequently withdrawn from their beats to meet other requirements, such as public order duties and meeting shortfalls of relief officers (Brown and Iles, 1985; see also Jones, 1980). The position has not improved since then. In our study, many CBOs complained at being withdrawn from their beats, often at short notice and without regard to community commitments (such as attending NW meetings) into which they might have already entered. This was less of a problem in Gwent, where all except two CBOs told us that they were never withdrawn from their beat. By comparison, in the Metropolitan Police District, a majority of CBOs told us that withdrawal from their beats was a significant problem. This appears to be most serious in the inner-city areas (where almost all CBOs complained) and, more generally, whenever relief officers are prevented from working overtime to make up staffing shortfalls. When relief officers are subject to overtime restrictions, CBOs are, as one put it, 'a reservoir of re-deployable people'.

Disruption of this kind was also said to be an increasingly serious problem in Avon and Somerset, where in one sub-division, for example, the number of CBOs was halved in order to make up shortfalls in the relief. The disruption caused to the work of beat officers was always a point of contention. In quantitive terms, whilst a few CBOs were highly susceptible to withdrawal to other duties because of their specialist skills (such as driving), most officers agreed that withdrawal was cyclical and overall was relatively infrequent (a few times a month was the most common). None the less, for beat officers, redeployment to other activities represented a lack of commitment to CBO work by the force, disturbed their own relationships with the community, and generally lowered their morale. The following quotations from CBOs are representative of the concerns expressed:

*Gwent*
(ex-CBO) I gave up being a [CBO] because I found that type of policing is not recognized by anyone other than the people out there. The people out there loved me, loved what I was doing. The Job didn't. They didn't like it at all because, while I was out there talking to people and solving their problems, they kept calling me away to other people's areas. . . . I was doing my school visits, going to community council meetings, patrolling the area on foot: to me, that was my job. But to my bosses – come and do this, come and do that. . . . I got to the stage where I was spending no time at all in my area; I was always away and it depressed me. That's why I asked to come away from it.

I am pulled off my beat a lot at the moment, especially with holidays and officers on leave. It is a shame that we are taken away but I don't think we can really argue about it, the job's got to be done. I'm in uniform: I haven't got [CBO] on my arm.

*Avon and Somerset*
I am very, very disgruntled at the moment, extremely disgruntled. We all have our moans and groans, policemen are prone to that, but since the scheme was introduced, the first day it was introduced in matter of fact, throughout the force and you have probably heard it before, the CBO system was brought in and right from the word go it was said that a community beat officer was never ever going to man the switchboard, never ever going to work nights, or do anything such like without express authority of the person in charge of the sub-division. Right from the word go we were standing in and just being used really for that sort of purpose, just standing in all over the place when somebody was off sick, somebody on leave.

Q: What are you doing now?
A: I *should* be walking my own beat as a [CBO]. But in reality, certainly this year, the situation's got worse and worse in that a [CBO] should be on his beat every single day but I've rarely been up on my beat. I've been pulled out of it certainly in the region of 75 per cent of the time, perhaps even 80 per cent.
Q: How do you feel about the situation at the moment?
A: It's very frustrating. Personally I'm sick to death of it. I've made various comments to my sergeant and inspector but it just seems to be getting worse. I'm allegedly a [CBO] . . . but I doubt if I've been on my beat now for the last two weeks. You tend to get a lot of shrugging of shoulders by everybody. They tend to sympathize. But I feel that I'm really only a [CBO] in name only. It just isn't working, it just isn't working at all.

*Metropolitan Police*
I get pulled off my duties a lot. Saturday I'm on aid to Trooping the Colour in Central London so I'll be off there. The Saturday following that I'm also up there again for Trooping of the Colour. This last Saturday I was on the Muslim demo, Westminster Bridge, stuck there. I've done football; I mean the week previous to this I've done football, I was at Wembley twice in the week, first for the Cup Final, [and then the] England v Chile

game. And it does really depress me, it does, it really gets to me. I think we do far too much of it as CBOs. It is very difficult, very difficult to get any sort of rapport going on that beat.

The [CBOs] have got to put down a schedule of what they are going to work for the week, and they are available for anything that comes up. So if a [CBO], which happened quite recently, had arranged to go to his Tenant's Association meeting that evening at half past seven, the day before he was informed that he was required to attend let's say a football match, and apparently he said to the sergeant, 'Well, you know I'm supposed to be at a tenant's meeting tomorrow night', 'Pity, you're required for aid'. So really and truly that has only got to happen three or four times and the guy says 'to hell with it I might as well be on relief, at least then I know what I'm doing; I'm doing either early turn, late turn or night shift'. And that is what we are killing [CBOs].

In justifying these practices, senior officers told us that personnel were 'put where they are most needed' or, quite bluntly, that 'the relief comes first'. A senior officer responsible for CBO work in Avon and Somerset reflected the views of many others when he explained that CBOs were called off their beats because 'the bobby on the beat saying "hello" is doing nothing and with the resources problem being as it is, we can't afford that any more'.

CBOs were expected to be available, therefore, not simply for 'aid' requirements (major crowd control or safety or security situations) but also to supplement shortfalls in the relief. And, as CBOs were quick to point out, police priorities did not operate in reverse: no one was called in to replace CBOs away for temporary absence, CBO beats could be left uncovered for substantial periods, and, in one case no efforts had been made to replace a CBO who had resigned because, according to a senior officer, no one had noticed the shortfall for over a month! However it is viewed, therefore, it is clear that other claims always outweigh those of community beat work, which still ranks lowest in police priorities, alongside training.

In his report arising out of the Brixton disorders, Lord Scarman (1981) made clear that effective beat policing depended upon improved training and supervision and on effective integration into the mainstream of operational policing. We shall deal with general issues relating to training in Chapter 7, and confine our remarks here to training with specific reference to the needs of community beat work. The general need for training for CBO work is well understood. Unlike relief policing of a fire-brigade kind, community beat policing involves relationships with the public rather than encounters, requires officers to establish long-term rather than fleeting connections with the community, and puts a premium on the resolution of problems, not just their containment. Such policing demands the development of attitudes and the acquisition of skills not conventionally needed by officers dealing with 'incidents' rather than community issues. The general problem with training for CBO work can be summed up simply: none is specifically provided. Beat officers time and again drew attention to the evils of a system which did not give them training in negotiating and communication skills, and which, furthermore, failed to explain the objectives of beat policing. The consequence for some officers was a lack of confidence in dealing with members of the public, the avoidance of situations where they might be called upon to speak, especially to gatherings of people, and a sense of insecurity about whether they were 'doing the job right'.

> When I first took on a [community] beat, I didn't really know what I was getting into and I asked for a job definition, and there isn't one. There wasn't then and there isn't now.

> Many constables don't want to be [CBOs] because they don't like having to go along to meetings, having to stand up and talk to people. I don't think they are prepared for it. It is not something they see as part of their job having to go to tenants' association meetings and having to talk to a group of thirty or forty people.

The problems in question – officers going out on patrol without clear objectives in mind, the lack of practical on-the-job training and the absence of training in skills essential to the proper discharge of beat policing – were all identified more than twenty years ago by a Home Office working party (Home Office, 1967b), were clear to constables and were apparent to some senior officers. These senior officers sought to minimize the problems where they could by selecting officers who they considered 'suitable' for CBO work. Even if this policy were considered appropriate, however, it could not be routinely implemented because of the unwillingness of officers to volunteer for CBO work. In all forces, to a greater or lesser extent, senior officers were forced to press-gang individuals into CBO work in order to make up staffing shortcomings. Thus, in our research samples, 38 per cent of CBOs in the Metropolitan Police District, 39 per cent in Avon and Somerset, and 55 per cent in Gwent, reported that they had not volunteered for their posting.

In some cases, 'press-ganging' was hardly appropriate to describe the process because some officers are sent to beat work as a *punishment* ('I was given the chief's catapult; sent here as a punishment', 'After a series of complaints about me on relief, I was consigned here [to CBO work]'). This meant also, in certain instances, the appointment of higher ranks to positions of responsibility for CBO work in which they had no belief. Thus, in one Avon and Somerset area, a CBO summed up the views of his colleagues about the new community involvement sergeant, who had been put in charge of CBO work, as follows: 'He quite openly thinks that community involvement is a pain in the arse, a waste of time and CBOs are a bunch of wasters. What's the point of having him there?'

The collective effect, therefore, in the absence of targeted selection and training procedures, was a system which heavily trusted to luck. Isolation from mainstream policing continues to be a problem in the Met. and Avon and Somerset but less so in Gwent, where CBOs are much more integrated into the reliefs. Although it liberated a few officers by giving them operational autonomy to work creatively in pursuance of community policing principles, in the case of most officers – as we shall see – it exacerbated loneliness, aimlessness and resentment.

## COMMUNITY BEAT OFFICERS: THEIR STATUS AND MORALE

Despite considerable efforts of management to foster its image, community beat policing is highly unpopular among constables. This was recognized in the Scarman Report (1981), where it was argued that community work was secondary in the eyes of many officers on the ground: in other words, it was not simply at the policy level that CB work was marginalized but also at an ideological level within the Metropolitan Police. In our research, we did encounter a handful of officers who reported a strong commitment to such work and who appeared to derive substantial job satisfaction from working within the community. In general, however, community beat work is considered by officers to be boring, unglamorous and disconnected from 'real' policing. Many officers, especially in urban areas, said that they did not want any closer involvement with a community which would give them 'hassle' and make their presence unwelcome. Younger officers want to band together in the reliefs where the camaraderie and *esprit de corps* reinforce a sense of mission and worth, and provide mutual support at times of boredom or crisis. Policing is seen as a collective effort directed towards the restoration of law and order rather than an individual task concerned with servicing the expressed needs of the community (Holdaway, 1983; Policy Studies Institute, 1983). The inability to fill community beat posts with committed volunteers is, therefore, a problem endemic to all three forces we examined.

No consistent policy designed to address this problem has been pursued and in some areas an air of desperation surrounded those responsible for CBO deployment. There was little talk of long-term commitment to a community, even though we were constantly told that an officer became effective on a beat only after working it for two to five years. Indeed, people were induced to become CBOs in some areas on the basis that it would be a one-year posting. Analysis of our research sample demonstrates the relatively high turnover rate to which community beat work is susceptible, most markedly in London. Thus, whilst one-fifth of Avon and Somerset and Gwent CB officers had been in the post for less than a year at the time of interview, this was true of over one-third of London CB officers. Moreover, officers were not necessarily selected on the basis of their personal qualities, some even being sent there as a discipline measure. Instead, officers were accepted for CB work even where it was known that their motivations were not positively directed toward community policing ideals or even where they appeared to be unsuitable. In the Met., for example, a number of officers (one-fifth of the volunteers) used a spell in CB work to study for promotional examinations, much to the annoyance of dedicated CBOs:

It seems to be a haven for people who want to study for the sergeants' exams; senior officers are always saying 'we don't want [CBOs] in that office that are there to study' but it still happens, we are just about to lose two who have passed the sergeants' and one bloke has transferred so we have had about four vacancies which are now filled, quite amazingly really, but again we've got prospective sergeants for next year's exam. They say one thing and another thing is done: I don't know whether it's political or what. The police can say the beat is filled no matter what proportion of the duty is going to be spent out on the street, sorting out the problems, or what proportion is going to be spent studying.

In no force, however, was the shortfall in CBOs made up by sufficient volunteers whatever their motivations. Management response in each force, with different levels of success, was to resort to compulsory transfer.

In Avon and Somerset and the Met. this policy did not find favour with any officer to whom we spoke. Feelings of dissatisfaction ranged from 'moaning and groaning' to officers harbouring 'bitter resentment'. It was routine for CBOs to describe themselves as 'pressed' officers, as having been 'lumbered' with a beat, or as having been 'put there'. Thus, when asked whether they had volunteered for their present post, officers often replied in the following way: 'It was a case of "volunteer or else you are going to be one"'; 'I am a pressed man'; 'I didn't volunteer. Definitely not. I was told to do it for a year' (Avon and Somerset officers) or as an officer from the Met. put it more cryptically, 'I was volunteered. In this job, you are volunteered.'

Although the policy of conscription was also deployed in Gwent, we found little sign of resentment among CBOs there, who generally viewed the experience in more positive terms. Although officers in the Met. assumed that a CBO posting in 'green and grassy districts is like gold dust and there's a queue a mile long', environmental attractions (which were equalled in much of Avon and Somerset) do not provide an explanation for the generally happier frame of mind of Gwent officers. What seems to have occurred, according to CBOs there, is that the positive features of beat work have become part of policing *culture* in Gwent. The virtues of CBO work are constantly broadcast, it is seen as an essential experience ('anybody who is anybody in Gwent police has been a beat officer'), and officers do not regard it as an unattractive or marginal part of policing. Several officers told us that being selected for CBO work was an accolade not, as in other forces, a punishment: 'I think you've got to be thought of to be a pretty good bobby to be asked to be a [CBO]. They are not going to ask anybody who doesn't work.'

The result was that in general beat postings were able to be filled in Gwent without the arm-twisting that characterized the other two forces, and officers were markedly more content than their counterparts elsewhere.

The status of the CBO in Gwent is closely connected with views held about beat work by relief officers there. All Gwent CB officers to whom we spoke felt that relief officers viewed community beat work positively or in the same way as relief work. Among relief officers themselves, criticisms of beat work were infrequent and muted, and tended to be related to the problems of the relief rather than to the characteristics of beat work itself. Thus, relief officers might describe CBO work as 'a bit of a luxury' because 'we are short of officers on the shifts', rather than decrying the value of working with the community. When asked about CBO work itself, relief officers, even in inner-city areas of Gwent, often spoke in positive terms: 'it is of tremendous value', 'it's important', and 'an excellent system' were typical comments. Relief officers generally said that there was no distinction drawn between relief and community beat officers: 'We don't regard [CBOs] as different'; 'We think the residential beat officers are the same as us: we don't differentiate'; 'I don't see us as being all that different really'.

By comparison, beat work and CBOs themselves are held in low esteem by relief officers in the Met. and Avon and Somerset, and CBOs tend in consequence to have a poor self-image. Relief officers routinely described beat work as mundane, and involving 'rubbish' that was 'bordering on the social worker side of things' or plainly 'irrelevant to policing'. The standard representation of beat work involved officers wandering about aimlessly, drinking cups of tea with old people, and divorced from the 'needs' of the area. CBOs in turn were usually seen as 'deadbeats', officers who were 'prematurely retired', and unwilling to help out when the need arose. Comments of the following kind typified relief officer views:

*Avon and Somerset*
I would say that the attitude in the police force is that community policing is a waste of time.

I don't believe that they enjoy being policemen because, as far as I'm concerned, they have ceased to become policemen. I know a lot of the CBOs think it's a complete and utter waste of time as well.

*Metropolitan Police*
They are not at the sharp end. They tend to disappear, if you like.

There's a joke that if your radio doesn't work, you've got a [community] beat radio, which generally means that [CBOs] don't answer them.

It is hardly surprising, therefore, that, unlike their Gwent counterparts, the overwhelming majority of CBOs in Avon and Somerset (80 per cent) and in the Metropolitan Police District (88 per cent) reported that community beat work was viewed negatively by relief officers. Lying behind this is a social reality about which many relief and beat officers are agreed: that being a CBO *does* involve 'rubbish' work (see Grimshaw and Jefferson, 1987, pp. 77–83). 'Rubbish' in this context is less indicative of issues such as parking, noise and stray dogs, which are usually referred to as 'grief', and more with the chores of policing: updating keyholder cards, serving summonses, taking statements about criminal offences which are unlikely to be cleared up. Indeed, relief officers sometimes value CBOs precisely because they relieve them of such 'rubbish'. As one Avon and Someset officer put it:

They do work for us basically, in that if they weren't there we'd end up doing the work they do, which is a lot of the everyday summonses, warrants, fixed penalties, enquiries, statements. . . . They take away a lot of the mundane work.

In describing their own work as involving 'rubbish', therefore, CBOs are not simply internalizing the negative attitudes held about them by relief officers; their evaluation of their work reflects the use that is made of them by the relief and the uninspiring character of some of the tasks they are required to perform.

The morale of CBOs and their commitment to their beats inevitably reflected these system-wide pressures. Those officers who had selected CBO work because they were committed to personal contact with the public tended to have very high job satisfaction. The universal expression of contentment among Gwent CBOs ('I am more than happy'; 'It suits my style'; 'I'd like to be left here for a number of years') found an echo in the other forces among officers who had dedicated themselves to CB work ('I'm happy as I am', Avon and Somerset officer; 'I will continue as a beat officer: I enjoy it', Metropolitan Police District officer). Officers enjoyed the autonomy that beat policing provided, not simply the escape from unsocial hours and shift work, but the freedom to run the beat in the way they thought best. As long as they were not withdrawn from their beat for other duties, these officers were able to establish sustained relationships with members of the local community. We found, as had Fielding *et al.* (1989) in their principal research site, that, where it appeared to work well, CBOs derived substantial personal benefits from relationships with local people in terms of job satisfaction and self-fulfilment:

> I run my beat because I want to and I enjoy doing it and hopefully that comes across to the people I police. I want to do it and I do care.

> Beat work I've found is far more interesting [than relief] because it is a communication with the community that I feel is essential to a police officer's health. I believe that the public want to have that rapport with the police.

The way that officers like this talked about their beats and the obvious pleasure they derived from being well known in the community, which we sometimes witnessed as we accompanied them on patrol, make it clear that beat policing can create enthusiasm in officers which is readily transmitted to the public.

At the other end of the scale are officers who suffer from low morale and low self-esteem and are awaiting a transfer. Many of those who were 'pressed officers' bitterly resent their time on beat work and are eager to get back to relief at the earliest opportunity. Some, of course, have been pleasantly surprised by their experiences and extend their tour of duty beyond the required period, but this was unusual except in Gwent. Indeed, only 44 per cent of CB officers in Avon and Somerset, and just 21 per cent in London indicated a desire to continue community beat work in the future. Altogether, almost one-fifth of CBOs in both of these forces had made arrangements to transfer from community beat work or, in a few cases, from the police service at the time of interview. Most of those who remained reported discontent and an intention to move at the first opportunity.

Generally speaking, press-ganged officers were intent on serving out their time as CBOs in a way which would require the minimum effort on their part consistent with avoiding drawing adverse attention to themselves in any way. This was particularly so in areas where police–public relations were fractured, and more generally, where police policies had backfired. This latter eventuality occurred in those cases where young officers, who often seek excitement, were put on beat work, and where senior officers 'sold' beat work as more exciting and rewarding than experience justified. All this was generally true of Avon and Somerset and the Met., where CBO work was marked by low morale and high staff turnover as reflected in the following typical comments:

*Avon and Somerset*
I've no intention of staying as a [CBO]. I'm on [community] beat now because I can't get off it really.

Hopefully, I'll be coming off here soon.

I'm very disgruntled.

*Metropolitan Police*
I would like to move on . . . but the problem is . . . that you find it hard to get experienced officers [in the inner-city subdivision]. The result is, I can't get off my beat because there is no one who will actually work the beat if I leave. So it's like being sent to the Russian front, you get here, it's very difficult as people have found to get away from here. . . . This beat was left vacant for about five months before I took it because it is regarded here as the worst beat, because of the area and negativeness and even the make-up of the area, being all council and that. People just don't want to do it, consequently the person who does it, finds it very difficult to get off it, like I applied to go into another squad and I got refused. It's very difficult to get away once you are here.

There are two beats on offer. They couldn't sell them here so they put it out as an order on the whole area for anybody who wants to come as a [CBO]. I saw the thing and I thought 'I'll apply for that' and then thought 'I am it!' They do advertising and there's no point in trying to sell something to somebody so when they get here it's not how it is; because you are only going to get a dissatisfied person.

## A failed policing initiative

The predictable result of all this was, in Avon and Somerset and the Met., a failed policing initiative. Senior officers, many of whom appear genuinely committed to community policing ideals, were caught in an unenviable dilemma. The image of CB work was so low that inadequate numbers of officers volunteered for postings, but forcing officers to accept assignments risked loss of morale and disgruntlement. Attempts to improve the image of CBO by presentational devices predictably led to disappointed expectations and further wastage. Where, as in some areas of Avon and Somerset, incentives were given to officers to become CBOs – typically a maximum secondment of one year, with for some, a driving course – the police, whilst plugging existing gaps, created a turnover treadmill. The effects of these policies were not confined to the police but, as our interviews with residents showed, were soon apparent in the community. People lost confidence in the idea of 'local' policing, thus making it more difficult for each new officer to gain local acceptance.

## THE WORK OF CBOs AND NEIGHBOURHOOD WATCH

Police officers tend to think of CB work as uneventful. Visiting schools, attending to non-urgent complaints, visiting the scene of a burglary to take statements of complaint, going out on general patrol, are seen as routine, often mundane, tasks. This makes CB work unattractive to many officers (see Chapter 6, below) who prefer to remain in, or to rejoin, the relief. Embedded in this conception of community policing, however, is a tension between crime-centred and service policing. This tension affects almost all CBOs. One of the reasons for this, of course, is simply a search for 'interesting' or 'exciting' work, conventionally associated with arresting criminals. In addition to this, officers feel they are given no credit for that which is not susceptible of measurement – 'getting along with the community' – and look for arrests to validate their own work and raise their standing in the eyes of the relief. Against this, however, is the tendency to avoid taking actions which will result in paperwork or lead to the disruption of relationships within the community. The way in which individual officers reconcile these conflicting tensions depends upon the extent to which they respond to external pressures and their own underlying value systems, as these officers make clear:

> The opportunities to go out and look for things the way you did on relief or on the Territorial Support Group just doesn't seem to be there as much. Sometimes I just sit there and think 'God, I haven't nicked anybody for weeks'.

> In the first year [of CB work] I put crime aside, any aspirations of going anywhere aside. I just concentrated on the community aspect. In the second year I just found myself doing [crime] and suddenly I realised that there's more important things to do than going along to meetings. . . . I thought, 'I want to be out doing things, running around, because the time may come when I can't do that'. So I went back into relief.

For the most part, however, CBOs involved themselves only marginally in crime, were not under pressure from senior officers to effect arrests, and spent their time developing links with the community. The success with which they did so varied dramatically from area to area, and from officer to officer.

Many officers told us that they had limited knowledge of the people in their areas, even after a considerable time spent in the locality. Many of the contacts they were required to make, such as dealing with complaints about noise, were not intended to be other than transitory, and few led to any continuing relationship. Moreover, in some urban areas police–public relations were poor in general and officers found it difficult to establish contact with members of the public. Overall, a characteristic of self-generated contacts (amply confirmed by the practices observed when we accompanied beat officers on patrol) is that they are confined to a few, select individuals in the community, usually shopkeepers, cafeteria owners, caretakers and similar types. These people were valued not simply because they offered refreshment opportunities (not an insubstantial benefit for a beat officer! ) but because of the knowledge which they possessed of the local community. The upshot was a very narrow range of contacts for many officers:

> I tend to talk mainly to people who have got their businesses there, to a few private people who are actually on committees and to anyone who has a problem.

> I always say good morning and good afternoon to people, but

we tend to try to talk more to the shopkeepers because they are obviously aware of the people in the area.

A similar pattern prevails in respect of neighbourhood watch. As is already apparent, CBOs in Gwent had little to do with NW. They had few schemes in the force area and made no efforts themselves to initiate new schemes. In the other forces, although officers' commitment to NW varied considerably, their contacts heavily focused upon NW co-ordinators rather than ordinary members of schemes. Officers reported that they tried to make contact with the co-ordinators 'once or twice a month', but many admitted that actual contacts were often less frequent, sometimes for understandable reasons:

> I'll explain my part in NW. I mean I'm the contact. I don't see them as much as I should do, I readily admit that. I should be seeing them, my co-ordinators, every couple of weeks or so but I just. . . . It's such strange hours. Like today I'm eight–four. It's nice hours; I sort of get up in the morning to be in work at eight and be home by four. But all the people who run the watch schemes of course are workers themselves, and so you miss them. And they don't see you out and about of course during the day, so when I do see them they say 'Oh haven't seen you for ages', you know. I mean they're a bit uppity about it.

This tends to be reinforced at NW meetings which are often attended only by co-ordinators. The picture of public interest in NW which emerged in Chapter 4 was amply confirmed by CBOs, who told us of poorly attended meetings following the initial launch, with, after a while, meetings being abandoned altogether in many areas. Whilst these meetings could be used to give people the latest crime figures – the main purpose of them so far as CBOs were concerned – they did little to deepen officers' knowledge of their beat area:

> Normally, I'll only meet co-ordinators regularly. At a meeting it's only co-ordinators, it's not everybody from the neighbourhood watch. So it's like, I could talk to members in the street and I wouldn't even know if they are part of my NW.

> With NW meetings, you only seem to get the people who volunteered in the first place.

The shortcomings of NW as a vehicle for establishing police–public relations arises principally because, as we have seen, the official emphasis on crime is not shared by most communities. After an initial flush of enthusiasm, schemes tend to founder and no amount of effort on the part of the police will reinvigorate dead schemes. But this further narrows the range of contacts that many officers have, seriously limits the value that they can bring to the community or derive from it, and further contributes to the isolation and disenchantment of officers who may have started beat work with high aspirations.

As a footnote we should add that some officers in all forces were themselves sceptical of the value of NW or in a few cases ignorant of its existence in their areas, and sought to carry out community policing ideals through other methods. For some, this was a response to public concerns about 'surveillance' and 'spying for the police', and for others it was a recognition of the inadequacy of crime as an organizing framework. The following Avon and Somerset officer, for example, who was regarded by everyone we spoke to as a dedicated community officer, talked about NW in these terms:

> When I speak to my bosses I call them neighbourhood watch groups and I speak to my residents as resident or community groups. It's important that I distinguish that because they do not like the image of neighbourhood watch. It's the image of the old woman sitting behind her curtain, peering out, making notes of cars driving past and everything else, which I don't believe would work anyway. Neighbourhood watch in itself is useless. If you just have individual people in the streets keeping an eye on what is going on, it doesn't help the community. If you can actually get the community actually working together with each other on a certain problem, then you are already half way there in beating it.

None the less, this attitude was not typical and CBOs were expected to provide support for existing NW schemes and (except in Gwent) to encourage the development of new ones. To what extent were they successful in this, and how did they go about their task?

## Official success and practical reality

It soon becomes apparent that there is a major and widening gulf between official representation of NW and ground level reality. According to government claims, as depicted in Chapter 1, NW is a story of rising success: once founded, the idea of NW captured the public imagination and the number of schemes grew rapidly throughout the 1980s. In August 1989, the Home Office minister John Patten described NW as 'an unstoppable movement' and linked the growth in schemes with crime statistics that suggested a reduction in property crime. However, in 1990, when statistics showed a record increase in recorded crime, Mr Patten had little to say about NW, concentrating instead on blaming victims for failing to protect their property (*Guardian*, 20 December 1990), a line he continued to follow on release of figures showing a massive rise in recorded crime during 1990 (*Guardian*, 28 March 1991). Although official figures sometimes distinguish between police forces, NW is implicitly depicted as having universal appeal, to be of equal value to poor as well as rich areas, the inner city as well as suburbs, estates as well as villages. The official picture, then, is one of rapid growth, comprehensive dispersal and reduced crime rates.

This view is emphatically not shared by the police themselves, although their actions do contribute to the maintenance of the successful image put forward by the Home Office. At a formal level, official policy requires that a substantial proportion of households in an area be members before a scheme can be accepted. This proportion appears to be 60 per cent of households (Smith, 1984). We found no senior officer responsible for NW organization who claimed that this recommended level of participation could be met. Commonly, officers said that the police would accept a figure of 25 per cent or less at launch and that no effort would be made to monitor membership levels after that point. The 'number of households covered' by NW in official figures must, therefore, be a substantial overestimate.

Whilst official figures speak of growth, senior officers responsible for the administration of NW speak of the collapse of schemes. In one area of the Met., for example, the officer responsible plotted the mortality rate of schemes on force area maps. These showed that of the thirty-two existing and five proposed schemes in mid-1986, only ten remained 'active' by the end of 1988. Other officers did not attempt to assess the real state of affairs, but their views were fully in line with this picture, as the following two examples from the Met. show:

Q: How many NWs do you have?
A: There are 110 schemes.
Q: How many of these would you describe as active?
A: Difficult to say. I would certainly be very surprised if half of them were active in the sense that people were talking about NW and holding regular meetings and actually doing things other than putting a sticker in their window and receiving a newsletter periodically.

Q: How many NWs do you have?
A: I've got fifty-seven.
Q: How many of these are active?
A: The active ones out of fifty seven are about twelve or thirteen, as low as that; so you are talking about 25 per cent.

In Avon and Somerset by contrast, senior officers generally put forward a more optimistic view, even if they accepted that they had no hard and fast figures, and did not monitor schemes in this way. While they accepted that many schemes failed, they wished to emphasize the positive aspects of NW and the numbers of new schemes (forty to fifty) established each month. In both forces, however, it is obvious that these private estimations of NW do not feed into the official figures. The bureaucratic imperative requires the reporting of new schemes with nothing being said about failed schemes. As one senior officer in London told us, when reporting the number of schemes in his area to force headquarters, 'You think of a number and double it!'

Police knowledge of inactivity levels of schemes is even greater at the level of the community beat officer. In both Avon and Somerset and the Met. officers reporting large numbers of active schemes were few indeed. Enthusiastic co-ordinators had in a few cases maintained schemes for many years. In Avon and Somerset, for example, one co-ordinator serviced thirty-four schemes centred on one village, and five main co-ordinators kept fifty-one schemes active in another village. Less impressive levels of success were achieved in other areas in both forces. In general, however, CBOs reported high levels of mortality, as the following illustrations show:

*Metropolitan Police*
On paper we have six schemes I think, of which one is active.

We have four schemes, but in only namesake really. They are inactive.

Neighbourhood watch looks good and works on paper. In an area like this, I would stick my neck out and say it doesn't work. I've got on my beat, I've got five NWs. If a senior officer said to me 'How many schemes have you got on your beat?', I'd say 'Five, sir', and if they then said 'How many have you really got?' I'd say 'None, sir'.

I have about twenty-eight schemes and about half of them are not active at all. The other half it varies. There are three or four that are quite active. Some more that are quite active if anything happens, and there is a number, of course, where people just are not interested at all.

*Avon and Somerset*
I have about nine schemes on my patch. They are mostly pretty passive. Four of the nine are quite active I should say.

I have about thirty-five schemes, probably no more than three or four of them are active.

There are officially seven schemes I'm responsible for but they are not going. For want of a better word I'd say they were dormant, all of them.

When questioned as to how they defined a scheme as 'active' or not, officers almost invariably reported that a scheme was considered active if it showed *any* sign of life beyond the existence of signs and stickers. This could be constituted by, for example, an occasional newsletter, meetings of residents, or contact between co-ordinators and the police (cf. Mayhew *et al.*, 1989). On this basis, it is clear that a large proportion of schemes on Home Office and police lists are effectively dead. Doubts expressed about the validity of official figures (see, for example, 'Home Office inflated watchdog figures', *The Observer*, 27 August 1989) are, therefore, wellfounded. A counting system which simply adds new schemes to existing totals, and does not remove schemes which have collapsed or are wholly inactive, fails to reflect what is happening in the real world and increases cynicism among those who have direct responsibility for the administration of neighbourhood watch. As one officer put it,

I think the, sort of, shall we say 'management' here are aware it's a flop really. I think so, from the sort of reactions you get. But I think at the end of the day obviously very, very senior management say 'we will have neighbourhood watch', so they've got to basically cater to their requests.

We can offer no 'true' count to pit against the official figures. The evidence clearly demonstrates, however, that the official picture massively overrepresents the number of schemes, that this is known to senior officers responsible for NW, and that the reality at constable level is even worse.

Whatever the official rhetoric, the police are under no illusions about the appeal of NW to certain groups in society and its lack of attractiveness to others. For the police, NW was not designed to appeal to the poorer sections of society and they hold out no real prospects for anything approaching a comprehensive coverage. Some senior officers told us that they were using NW to improve the police image rather than as a crime prevention device:

I've recently put a watch into somewhere that didn't have any crime. You might well ask why I did it, why didn't I tell them I don't need it. We're very much into wanting the public to like us, because we lost face with the public at the turn of the 60s through the 70s, and we have got a long way to draw it back. If your average member of the public comes to us and wants something, if we can give them something that won't cost a fortune that makes them think the police are a good lot, then they're going to speak up on our behalf. It's good P.R. to give it to them . . . so we've eased people's minds, we've gained friends and supporters. It's good P.R.

More important than this, however, is the general police system of values, apparent since the formation of the 'new police' in the early decades of the nineteenth century (see Silver, 1967; Storch, 1975; Scraton, 1985) which divides society into the rich and the poor, and the working class into the 'roughs' and the 'respectables' (see Reiner, 1985). These loose divisions provide the police with working rules that can be applied to the areas they think are suitable for NW. Police efforts then become largely directed to establishing schemes in areas where support can be almost guaranteed or where there is unlikely to be overt, hostile opposition. For the police, 'community' is generally associated with the white, middle-

class, property-owning section of society living out a quiet, pros-
perous and law-abiding life. Their conception of NW is that it will
have appeal to such communities, but little appeal elsewhere:

Q: Do you encounter difficulties in establishing schemes?
A: You always face the argument that neighbourhood watch
seems to be, because of its nature, seems to be aimed at
property-owning people more than anything else.
Q: Do you think there is any substance in that?
A: Oh yes, I think it's true. I think the 'haves' rather than the
'have-nots' prefer to have neighbourhood watch. The 'have-
nots' see no use in it.

Neighbourhood watch is all right in some areas. I don't like to
talk about class, but owner-occupier country. People who own
their own houses, pay their rates and taxes, and presumably
spend quite a lot on their houses too.

The people who are going to join a scheme are a certain type
of person, the more respectable and the people that would assist
the police.

These broad conceptions have direct consequences for the distribution of NW schemes. We found, as had Sampson *et al.* (1988),
that NW can foster divisions between estate dwellers and non-
estate dwellers, thereby helping to 'reinforce stereotypical images
of crime-ridden estates' (p. 486). In the cities, whenever officers
spoke about NW the contrast was invariably between residential,
property-owning areas and 'estates', as in the following examples:

The actual policing where I am, with the council estates, I don't
feel that this works, NW. I found the most interest we've got has
come from the privately owned properties where if people get
burgled, apart from their household insurance, it's up to them
to pay for physical repairs to houses. Whereas on the council
estates, if the door gets smashed open the council repair it; if
the window is broken the council repair it, and people don't take
so much pride in their actual living conditions, than owner-occupied houses. Most of the people on the estate are generally
unemployed and all got their fingers in different pies. All of
them know people from whom they can buy a bit of stolen stuff
from and all of them can sell a bit of stolen stuff; so to have a
neighbourhood watch in an estate like that is total taboo.

To be very honest with you I don't pay too much attention to NW at the present time because for me – I'm not getting any feedback from anyone so whether it's working or not I really don't know. Also the first meeting I ever went to which was this, you read in the papers it's all predominantly white, middle class and that's what happened, it's all white, middle class. But that's just the street it was on. All the villains won't have NW because they're the ones doing all the crime, they sort their own problems out.

I find that on council estates there isn't that many schemes because of their attitude towards the police. They think they will be considered police informers. There is the situation where, because they live on these estates where there are criminals and everything else and they are frightened that if they start ringing the police and trying to form something like this, we're not going to be able to be there all the time and they are frightened that things might happen to them.

In police culture, council estates harbour 'criminals' and 'villains' who have every interest in shutting out agencies associated with the force so that they can continue their life-styles without interference. Police value systems of this kind were underpinned in some areas by their failure to incorporate estates into NW schemes and by the lack of friendliness towards them displayed by residents. Police conceptions of the rough element of society had, therefore, some empirical reality, although officers too readily equated a lack of friendliness with villainy. But officers did not require validation for their views: time and again we were told that there 'was no point' in trying to launch a scheme in estate areas because these were known to be inappropriate. In this way, whole sections of the black community of London and Bristol were written off by local officers as unfit for neighbourhood watch or other community-based policing initiatives. This was neatly illustrated when, after an officer described a scheme in a middle-class enclave surrounded by working-class communities, we asked whether NW would be spread outwards to cover adjacent areas and he replied, 'No, it's them that the scheme is protecting members from.'

## THE VALUE OF NW: THE POLICE VIEW

Whatever the rhetoric about beat officers 'getting along with the community', there can be no real doubt of the importance in official policy of the intelligence-gathering function of patrol officers. The Home Office working party which stimulated moves to uprate the status of beat work, for example, laid most emphasis upon the acquisition of criminal intelligence and its transmission to other force officers (Home Office, 1967a). John Alderson, often credited with supplying the most fully worked out theory of community policing, also portrayed the beat officer as someone whose job it was to penetrate the community (Alderson, 1979). Similarly, Brown, a researcher closely associated with official thinking, whilst asserting that the job of the CBO was 'firmly rooted in sustained community relations with a primary emphasis on prevention' added that the CBO 'provides an essential source of information – the police blood stream – for other arms of the service' (Brown, 1979, p. 1051). Bearing in mind the way officers in general evaluate community beat policing, it is quite clear that the principal instrumental value for the police of neighbourhood watch is its ability to generate crime information. It cannot be assumed that the broad failure of CBOs to engage with residents and the concentration of their efforts on a select few – co-ordinators, shopkeepers, estate managers, caretakers – results in the non-production of criminal intelligence. That is an issue which needs to be separately tested. In this section, we examine the extent to which NW is 'successful' in this respect.

The first point to notice is that some beat officers, albeit a small minority, see their job in crime-oriented terms. On occasions this involves the officer in personally seeking out arrests. This will be very rare, however, because the more an officer focuses upon pro-active and interventionist policing methods, the more difficult it will be to gain a measure of acceptance in the community, the more information will dry up, and, in consequence, the fewer the opportunities will be to utilize such policing methods. (As one CBO put it, 'You can upset a lot of people arresting the son of one of your area co-ordinators for a minor infringement which could be dealt with by a good bollocking or telling his father.') Crime-oriented officers tend to concentrate, therefore, upon information gathering. This can be undertaken by befriending people in the community, gaining their confidence, and waiting for useful material to be offered or inadvertently passed, as the following officers make clear:

> A [CBO] is a person who has got to establish himself in the community, as far as I'm concerned. He's got to get to know the people and gain their trust, and from that he can glean very valuable information for other officers.

> Some days I spend the majority of my time just talking to shopkeepers, gleaning any information. They mostly don't realize they're giving you the information as you talk to them.

There was very broad agreement among both CBOs and relief officers that, insofar as it has any value at all, information acquired by beat officers was useful in facilitating operations already contemplated by other officers rather than directly initiating police action. Whilst, therefore, beat officers occasionally came by information from co-ordinators or other members of NW which produced a 'good arrest', their main value lay in easing the task of other officers. Thus they were able to facilitate the arrest of an individual sought by the police through their knowledge of the individual's habits and routines, and could provide officers with 'safe houses' from which observations could be conducted. The longer officers are attached to a single beat and the closer the knowledge of the community, the greater the value they have for other officers in these respects.

At its highest, therefore, beat work in which the officer is heavily integrated into community information networks could lend substance to the concerns of critics of officially-sponsored crime initiatives that they lead to greater control of the community, extending the reach of the criminal justice system and dispersing it (Cohen, 1979; Mathieson, 1980). A specific criticism of NW has been its information-gathering power, which can be used as a means of breaking down and penetrating community resistance:

> Such intelligence gathering has an increased importance in the context of the development of police collators, that is sophisticated, sometimes computerised, methods of collating routine information about people which officers pick up in the course of their duties, and which often consist of hearsay and other unverifiable material.
>
> (Gordon, 1984)

In this view, CBOs are not separate from other forms of policing, including pro-active and interventionist styles. Instead, they are an essential part of the police, not simply softening the public image of the police but a necessary adjunct which makes reactive policing possible and more effective. Whilst the potentiality of this policing model should not be glossed over, and whilst the effectiveness of CBOs in this respect will always be hard to detect ('The whole point of being a beat officer is that you don't get actively involved in the actual arresting of people; you try and keep out of sight when that happens'), there are very good reasons to believe that, as it currently operates, community beat policing is ineffective at this level.

The first observation to make is that many CBOs are neither crime-oriented nor particularly assiduous at gathering intelligence information. As we have seen, many are not volunteers and are beat officers for reasons which are more closely related to their personal career development than to overall policing needs. Many of those conscripted to beat work are simply concerned to serve out their term until they can get back to relief, move on to a specialist squad or retire. Conversely, many of those who are most dedicated to beat work are officers who have internalized community policing ideals relating to service, and have little belief or interest in the production of crime information through NW or otherwise. What other officers may see as 'mere PR' – talking to people in the community about their non-policing concerns, working with youth clubs, organizing 'events' and so forth – represents for these dedicated officers core policing activity in which the police are an ancilliary to the social services network. The scorn that is consistently directed at such officers by the relief ('He couldn't nick himself shaving', 'I bet you they couldn't even tell you the combination to the chargeroom door'), is a testimony to the fact that the priorities of many CBOs lie elsewhere than in intelligence gathering.

A second point is that, insofar as NW schemes are 'successful' in social terms, they are unsuccessful in police terms. Schemes, as we have seen, tend to take hold most strongly in white, middle-class, property-owning areas, which do not produce crime information of the kind which is valued by the police. The crime-centred representation of NW actually contributes to its demise. Crime is not a salient feature of most people's lives and quarterly crime figures presented to meetings of NW which demonstrate the 'crime-free' nature of the area confirm the sense that residents have that they should not be worried about crime. Conversely, in those areas of most interest to the police, NW is not established, beat officers often have little to do with the local community, and such crime information as is produced, is generated in traditional ways, namely individuals informing on each other for private more than public-spirited motives.

This links to a point constantly made by all beat officers, that the quality of the information provided by the general public is routinely low grade. Although there is some substance in the view that the denigration of the public so common among police officers is an assertion of police professionalism and the correctness of their judgements over those of citizens (Shearing, 1981b), there can be no doubt that the consistency of responses from officers of all ranges of experience in all areas of our study is eloquent testimony to the, in police terms, mundane nature of much information passed to the police. Altogether, over 80 per cent of CBOs in Gwent, over 70 per cent in Avon and Somerset, and some 60 per cent in London, rated the information given to them by members of the public as of little value, or as too general to be of any use; and, of the remainder, almost all officers in the three force areas agreed that useful information was offered only 'occasionally'. These are remarkable figures, given the reluctance of many officers to dismiss information ('No information is useless, but what I get is pretty trivial', Avon and Somerset officer). Part of this evaluation is based upon the willingness of members of the public to pass on 'gossip' and their unwillingness to provide formal statements as witnesses where their information is crime-relevant. So far as the police are concerned, there is an inadequate supply of good (crime-related) information, and what there is, is too little, too late and of questionable value:

> I find the people in the area very reluctant to 'phone the police with what they would think is non-useful information. They will 'phone up the next day and say 'at midnight last night, there was a prowler in my back garden', but that isn't any good to anybody. They should be 'phoning up at the time. It might be that there's nobody there and we don't find anybody, but the chance of finding anybody the morning after is nil.

> I should say 90 per cent of what you get told is of no use whatsoever to the police force. A lot of it is hearsay, a lot of it is

just general village talk about who is having whose wife, that sort of thing; no use to us whatsoever.

I pick up some information, not very much. I get some. You always pick up snippets of information, from talking to people. You pick up little snippets, but nothing really concrete. Nothing like someone who has witnessed something and says 'I will go to court and I will be a witness' because they won't.

Some of the people are very good. They do ring up if they think something's wrong, and you'll go down. All right, 99 times out of 100 it's nothing, but for the one time in 100, and even if it's one time in 1,000, if it turns out to be something, it's gotta be worth it. Having said that . . . I went to a call where a burglar had gone in through a top window, nicked some stuff. He's carrying a bag and a radio cassette and he's in the back garden, he can't get through the back gate, and the next door neighbour who is the landlord of this flat comes out and goes 'Er, can I help you?'. He said, 'Yeah, I can't get through the gate'. So he opened the gate for 'im, and about an hour later thinks [in silly voice] 'Oh! That was funny!' and rings us up, y'know . . . and he was NW! [laughs].

Crime-oriented officers are rapidly disillusioned by the quality of information generated through NW and, more generally, from the public. Officers draw a distinction between 'good crime' and 'rubbish'. Good crime includes both crimes of a serious variety committed by experienced villains (Policy Studies Institute, 1983) and also crimes such as burglary when these can be cleared up; if they cannot be cleared up, they are 'rubbish'. According to the police, the public have little or no knowledge of 'good class villains', and will not come forward with useful information that they might possess about serious local crime, because they do not want to get involved or are too frightened. As a result, information they are willing to pass on is either non-serious or non-crime matters, or is something which involves them personally. Information of this character is looked at sceptically by officers because of the questionable motives which produced it, as the following quotations make explicit:

Information is a load of crap to be honest. The fact that they've been ever so helpful, I wouldn't dream of giving the impression of anything else, whatever they tell me, I'll give my best serious

face and say 'Oh, it's great, thanks very much' because at the
end of the day they might come back with something good. It
ranges from 'He's having noisy parties' to car tax; the car tax
really is an old favourite . . . I think every time someone has an
argument with his next door neighbour they 'phone up here
and say 'He hasn't got a tax on his car', you know, things like
that.

We do have surveys every now and again to see what they think.
Unfortunately, we expect them to say street robbery or burglary
is their main concern, but it's always more to do with the
neighbour's car not being taxed. That's always coming up at
NW meetings. You're expecting them to be worried about the
bogus water board official and they're more concerned that
they're having to pay their car tax and their neighbour isn't.

The people who provide information from NW give us useless
information or they are the same people who used to contact
us anyway before: nosey parkers, busybodies, and vindictive
people, all of them providing low level information about low
level incidents.

Little of the information collected by CBOs was, therefore,
memorialized, and most of it was not passed on to the collator. The
lack of integration of CBOs into standard policing further marginalized the value of any data they did gather. In many areas
examined, we found a total lack of co-ordination between the
efforts of CBOs and other officers, so that relief officers were
ignorant of anything of value possessed by CBOs. The fractured
relationship between beat officers and their relief counterparts
makes the intelligence-gathering ideal unrealizable.

## CONCLUSION

Both in terms of official force policy and the public views of senior
officers, all three police forces studied embraced a service model
of policing, although only Avon and Somerset and the Met. saw
neighbourhood watch as an important vehicle for discovering
what the community wants and meeting its needs. All forces,
however, have had difficulty in translating these aspirations into
practical policies, with CBOs being everywhere a small minority
of constables. The proclaimed institutional commitment to beat

policing is called into question by the low priority accorded such work, seen in terms of the withdrawal of officers from beat work, the lack of training programmes, and the selection procedures forced on senior officers by the unattractiveness of beat work to the lower ranks. In general and with some outstanding exceptions, the two forces apart from Gwent have found it impossible to raise the status of beat officers or to raise their morale. The conscription system and the low morale of officers finds expression in work patterns that emphasize 'easing' behaviour (Cain, 1973) rather than constructive efforts to engage with the local community. Neighbourhood watch has proved an ineffective vehicle for overcoming these problems, encouraging in officers community links which are confined to co-ordinators, and serving to confirm officer's pre-existing views of the public as poor sources of crime information, the litmus test for most constables of any policing initiative.

Against this background, CBOs were sharply divided in their views as to the worth of NW. Leaving aside Gwent (where positive sentiments towards NW were often expressed by constables), we found some officers still committed to the principles of NW. In general they took the view that it brought benefits for the police in terms of good public relations and that it did, or might, provide a deterrent to potential burglars. Most, however, were unenthusiastic. They had seen many schemes fail and, despite considerable personal efforts on the part of some, had found substantial areas unresponsive to NW. In addition, many took the view that it was impossible to maintain public interest in most schemes after the initial impetus was lost. The constant turnover of staff among CBOs led to uneven and destructive policies, with, for example, established schemes failing because of the lack of commitment of a new CBO, and new CBOs losing their enthusiasm because of community resistance linked to a legacy of neglect by predecessors. In some areas, officers felt that force policy demanded a continued expansion of schemes; in other areas there was no such pressure on officers or they were resistant to it.

# Chapter 6

# Police culture: blue lights and black people

We have seen that whilst a few officers are dedicated to the ideals of community policing and to serving the needs of the community through the mechanism of neighbourhood watch, most officers have no desire to be involved with this kind of policing and have no specialist knowledge of or sympathy with the neighbourhood watch system. In this chapter we begin to explore why the majority of officers hold views which are opposed to community policing precepts, how they understand their social world, their own role in it, and the consequences for the communities they police.

Despite the organizational, hierarchical and bureaucratic structure of the police, the lower ranks retain considerable operational autonomy. In the police, discretion increases 'as one moves *down* the hierarchy' (Wilson, 1968, p. 7). Whilst the perspective and influence of management cannot be ignored (see Chapter 7, below), it is on the lower ranks that the attention needs to be focused. As Reiner put it,

> It is a commonplace of the now voluminous sociological literature on police operations and discretion that the rank-and-file officer is the primary determinant of policing where it really counts – on the street.

(1985, p. 85)

The range of studies to which Reiner adverts (see for example Banton, 1964; Skolnick, 1966; Bittner, 1967, 1970; Rubinstein, 1973; Cain, 1973; Manning, 1977, 1979; Chatterton, 1976, 1983; Holdaway, 1979, 1983; Ericson, 1982; Punch, 1983) and those which have appeared subsequently (see for example Jones, 1986; Grimshaw and Jefferson, 1987; Fielding, 1988b; Foster, 1989; Graef, 1989) amply confirm the importance of the powerful, if not monolithic, view of the lower ranks. It is to this occupational culture which we first turn in order to begin to explain widespread antipathy towards community policing and neighbourhood watch within the police. We then go on to explore the effects this culture exerts upon everyday policing.

## OCCUPATIONAL POLICE CULTURE

In the police world-view, society, ever-threatened by the forces of evil, is teetering on the brink of disorder and chaos, held in place only by 'the thin blue line'. Officers, who see themselves unequivocally on the side of right and good, place the threat of crime and political disorder at the centre of their image of society. Crime in this context is a serious infraction of the rules of civilized behaviour which merits firm condemnation and celerity of punishment. To effect this, officers want the core of policing to be aggressive, action-centred encounters with citizens. Whilst this is a characteristic of urban police officers, traces of it also appear in rural officers, though in a much more muted form.

### The blue light syndrome

Policing, in this view, is marked by speed, excitement, variety and uncertainty – 'the blue light syndrome' in canteen culture. A chase, going to potentially exciting calls, rushing to the aid of other officers who have requested urgent assistance, all provide experience of 'real' policing, as the following quotations from relief officers make clear:

Q: What do you like about the job?
A: Certainly the night-time activity. When you do nights, it gets exciting.
Q: What happens?
A: When there's 'urgent assistance' and you have to go somewhere fast, you shoot round in the car. That's one of the best bits about it.

Q: So what's so attractive about relief?
A: It's because you're never really sure what you're doing. It can be a real laugh all together. It can be exciting at times, if you don't know what is going to happen.
Q: What do you find exciting?

A:  Well, it's exciting if you get a call for assistance and there's a whole lot of you going down there. You don't know what you're going to find, and there's the camaraderie and that.

Q:  Why is relief work attractive to you?

A:  Well, it's the rushing around and all that; that does it for me.

Here, uncertainty and excitement are seen in positive terms, and outweigh what might be thought of as unattractive aspects of policing – danger and the possibility of physical assault. Far from being deterred by such eventualities, officers see these as increasing the sense of excitement and mission (Cain, 1973; van Maanen, 1974; Holdaway, 1983; Fielding, 1988b). Thus, after one officer was asked to explain why he preferred relief work to community beat and replied that 'the appealing aspect of shift work is that you are out on the streets', we pointed out that this was also true of community beat work; the interview continued,

> Yes, but statistically speaking, I mean you can get a murder happen at any time or a fire happen at any time, but it's going to be that the most punch-ups are going to be on a Friday night say; that is when you are going to get the adrenalin flowing, which you are not going to get walking around on a Monday morning.

If action of any kind is considered 'proper' policing, relief officers routinely said that the most enjoyable aspect of their work was arresting people. Time and time again, officers told us that authentic policing involved arrest:

> I enjoy arresting people, surveillance, that's what I happen to enjoy. I still get enthusiastic over arresting a good sort of burglar or mugger.

> I like getting out and getting amongst them. I get more satisfaction out of doing that, getting involved and arresting people, and that is what I see my job as.

> I can't call it a thrill, but the old adrenalin's going. You go to a call 2–3 o'clock in the morning, 'suspects on premises' and anyone would: the object is to get there fast. It's not the thrill of driving a car, flashing blue lights; it's just the opposite. You actually drive there without any lights, without being seen.

That's where the thrill comes, in actually catching someone worthwhile – that's what we are here for.

Against this representation of real policing, community beat work and the ideals of community policing were very unattractive. At its lowest, community beat work was constantly characterized as 'drinking cups of tea with old ladies', 'visiting schools and talking to children', 'attending meetings': activities which were not real police work. Community beat work was widely considered as something for 'older officers', perhaps desirable when 'working out your last few years', a 'nice job, semi-retirement, before retirement'. In terms of in-service experience, these images had some foundation in reality. Thus, in our sample, even discounting the initial probationary period (which may include short spells with community officers but is primarily served on attachment to the relief) we found a high proportion of officers with ten or more years' service in community beat work as compared to the relief (in Gwent, 86 per cent as against 25 per cent; in Avon and Somerset, 53 per cent as against 29 per cent; and in the Metropolitan Police District 20 per cent as against 11 per cent). Looked at in another way, in CB work there were no raw recruits; but in relief work on average there was a comparatively high proportion of officers of short standing: one-fifth of Avon and Somerset and Gwent officers and over one-third of London officers had two years' service or less.

Looked at overall, community beat policing was not attractive to most relief officers. This was much less true of Gwent, where CB work enjoyed a higher status, but even here 52 per cent of relief officers said that they did not wish to become community beat officers. In the Metropolitan Police District and in Avon and Somerset, by contrast, relief officers were almost universal in their rejection of CB work. Indeed, in London 96 per cent and in Avon and Somerset 87 per cent of relief officers interviewed said that they were not attracted to community beat policing and positively did not intend to apply for any such posting. The following quotations illustrate the sorts of response relief officers gave on this question:

Q: What is it about community beat work that doesn't appeal to you?
A: Basically the hours, the fact that I would have to walk all the time, and whilst I don't mind now and again listening to Mr

Smith whingeing about this, that and the other, I don't want to hear it all the time. I like driving the car; it's a fast response vehicle. To me it's exciting, . . . you know, you chase cars and that.

It's the sense of excitement which is attractive on relief. That goes hand in hand with the uncertainty of the job. I can tell you now, there is certainly no waiting list for [community beat]. It is rather an unexciting, uneventful form of policing.

The one who should be doing [community beat] has 20–25 years' service, and there's no one here like that in this station. I'm an *active* policeman.

I have spoken to some of the [CBOs] and it's something that I don't think will appeal to me. I prefer to be out doing general duties. . . . From what I have seen it is just going round schools and talking to kids, wandering around talking to the locals. I mean it's a bit too staid; I like the variety.

Community beat work did not, therefore, hold out the promise of real policing to most officers, even for those who accepted that CB work had a value for the police as a whole, as one Metropolitan relief WPC explains in the following interview extract:

Q: How are CBOs viewed within the police?
A: Some officers think they are a waste of time and effort.
Q: Why?
A: I don't know, because they are not. . . . They say they are a waste of time, they are not bringing in bodies [making arrests] . . . but they forget that we need the other side of it, a community policeman that can help get the public rapport up with us, because without them a lot wouldn't trust the police and they wouldn't come forward and the schoolchildren wouldn't have any respect for the police at all.
Q: Do you think the work of a CBO is of significant value?
A: Yes . . . many a time you get telephone calls from people who live on the estates that are having certain problems. You can chat to them for as long as you can, but they actually need a visit from a policeman. You know that it's not worthwhile sending a relief officer, so what you do is send round the [CBO] for that area. . . . It's jobs that aren't urgent but they still need a police presence.

Q: Have you ever thought about doing CB work yourself?

A: No. I don't feel I would enjoy it. I don't know why. I think it's because I enjoy being out on the streets and being involved in what is happening on the streets. . . . Basically, I think it's the adrenalin.

Not surprisingly, management is often unable to fill CBO vacancies with volunteers. One senior officer in the Metropolitan Police, who was concerned at the inability of the force to inculcate in officers the values of community policing, nevertheless understood the problems confronting policy-makers who might wish to move away from fire-brigade policing:

It's difficult to explain to someone who's never actually been involved in the police force. I think when you're young and you've started out on a police career, I think without exception recruits join the police force, as well as for all the other reasons, they would say in 100 per cent of cases they're looking for a bit of excitement, and I think many of them see that the possibility of going round in a police car to fast calls, getting there and arresting blokes in hooped jerseys with 'swag', taking them into the police station, it's almost orgasmic to them. Against that, looked at in the cold light of day, tea with an eighty-six year old granny comes very low down their scale of priority.

As Cain (1973) has pointed out, this image of relief policing as crime-oriented is tenaciously held by officers even though crime forms a very minor part of their working lives. Thus, in the United States, Reiss (1971) found that 80 per cent of calls were non-crime calls, and, in England, Punch and Naylor (1973) found that service calls in three Essex locations ranged from 50 to 70 per cent of calls (see also Holdaway, 1983; Heal *et al.*, 1985). Indeed, most policing is characterized by a lack of excitement: it is mundane, uneventful, and boring in the eyes of officers. Walking the beat can be very lonely, is often felt to be aimless, and is not likely to produce an exciting encounter:

It is very, very rare that you will be walking down the street on a night-time when you hear the burglar breaking the back window or see the burglar climbing up the drainpipe. It's never happened to me.

Many of the times you are walking the streets aimlessly, you know from six in the morning to two in the afternoon; it's very rare you are going to come across a crime.

Similarly, although relief work is depicted by officers as exciting, involving travelling by car or van, rushing from scene to scene, this is very rarely connected with criminal incidents and is much more often 'low-grade service work', as the following examples make clear:

> Once you have passed your driving course then you become a messenger. 'Would you go around and tell Mrs Smith we have found her dog?', 'Would you tell Joe Bloggs he's at court tomorrow?', 'Will you tell someone else we have found his car?'. So basically you race around the ground just giving out messages to people. You can't chat to people: you can allow people four or five minutes of your time because the person at the station is calling you up on the radio to deal with something else.

> The job of relief is to answer the calls, all the calls that come through to the station. A lot of these are very minor calls and a lot of time we get involved with delivering messages, doing court warnings and the like, which although necessary is time-consuming and not directly connected with police work a lot of the time.

The way in which officers conceptualized their jobs was usually a dialogue with the mundane reality, an attempt to come to terms with the routine without abandoning the myth of excitement. Relief work was attractive because it offered 'variety'. The unusual, atypical moments of excitement were given life in their characterization of the 'attractive' aspects of policing: these were, invariably, 'uncertainty', 'you never know what is going to happen next', 'when the wheel comes off, everything goes pear-shaped'. In this way, officers authenticate and instantiate the thrills they associate with real policing, deprive the mundane of importance, and provide a means of sustaining themselves as they go about their daily routines:

> There is a lot of just plodding around, I'll be quite honest with you but there is, like for instance yesterday it was raining, and just walking around, there was nothing going on, and you think what am I doing this job for you know! But then you think about the better times, the more exciting times where you know you

have a chase or you stop somebody that's wanted or you know basic everyday things, you deal with shoplifters, that sort of thing, it's all very interesting work. Maybe some people wouldn't think it was exciting.

## Servicing the relief or the community?

Whilst almost all Gwent and Avon and Somerset relief officers, and a majority of those in London, felt that there was value in community work, community beat work was generally looked upon favourably by reliefs only in terms of its contribution to servicing relief needs. Occasionally this is in the form of providing background information about suspected criminals or in supplying an address for use as an observation post, but more often it is in the form of discharging mundane tasks (such as serving warrants and notifying witnesses) that would otherwise fall to the reliefs, or providing a boost to the image of the force, as the following officer makes clear:

*Metropolitan relief officer*
The job of [CBOs] is to go round and be public relations officers, and be nice to people and walk the streets so they can't say: 'We never see a policeman walking the streets'. That's their job. And I think the rest of us should be in minibuses, going round responding to crime, and getting them and nicking them.

Understanding the job description in terms of action and excitement leads relief officers into a style of policing that contrasts sharply with that of those CBOs who are committed to the service ideal. Dedicated CBOs talk in terms which celebrate the value of symbolic presence, reassuring people by their presence and their accessibility. In this policing style, crime has a subordinate place:

My own view point is I don't go out there to get information on criminals and bring it back and deal with it. That's a very small chunk of it because basically the way I have seen it and the way it works, communities can deal with crimes themselves, they don't really need a police force as such. It's amazing how they can educate their own youngsters not to break into other people's houses.

Establishing relationships in the community, spending time talking to people, are seen in positive terms and contribute to a 'successful' day. And if work becomes wholly uneventful, officers may seek satisfaction in activities of a similar character, reinforcing the attributes of the job they have come to value:

> There is one thing in that it can get very lonely out there, walking around on your own. If I get the opportunity to walk with another [CBO] whether it's on an adjoining beat or opposite ends of the ground I'll do it just for the chance to talk, and have a look at their beat. So as much as possible I will pair up with other officers on the beat, and go out strolling, just for the case of chatting to someone for something different to do.

By contrast, relief officers who cling to the 'blue light syndrome' of policing, find difficulty in coping with walking around the beat, spending time uneventfully:

> Q: Is relief work in any way stressful?
> A: I suppose it is, but you don't notice it, you get used to it; especially here it is very busy. I suppose I find *not* doing anything more stressful than doing something. If you do night duty or station officer and nothing happens, that is more stressful than running around. (original emphasis)

To alleviate the stress of boredom we found, as had Cain (1973) and the Policy Studies Institute (1983), that relief officers would engage in pro-active work in order to foster the partial experience of authentic policing.

> I find I tend to have my own little personal objectives so I don't get bored. Like, not necessarily hassling a certain person, but I'll say: 'Right, let's get to know *him*; he's at it, whatever'. I'll stop him if I can and see what he's doing, see what he's about. Of an evening, prostitutes. If you want something to do of an evening, then you do observations on a prostitute and nick her, which only takes ten minutes to deal with. She'll be back on the street after that [laughs].

This 'machismo' culture is especially problematic for women police officers (Young, 1991). Whilst a majority of policewomen either enjoyed relief work ('Its like a big family on my relief. . . . Excellent', 'We're all friends, we're not just colleagues', 'I get a lot of support from my colleagues'), or did not express their complaints in terms of gender, some 40 per cent of women officers interviewed in the research spontaneously complained of being actively discriminated against as women or of being forced to tolerate negative canteen behaviour associated with masculine values. The emphasis by male relief officers upon masculinity and masculine values, reinforced by crude 'canteen-talk', was not lost on policewomen, as the following quotations make clear:

It's all a load of crap what [the relief] come in with. They would never, I mean sometimes some of the language that they use is so bad and so disgusting, I just sit there . . . I just sit there quietly unless it affects me. But sometimes when abuse has been turned on me I have turned round and said: 'You wouldn't say that at home to your wife, or if anyone said that to your wife you'd bloody hit them wouldn't you?' And it's true they would!

You get fed up sometimes when they take the mickey out of you, but you have to accept that you are here in a man's world, more of a man's world than most other jobs.

As the Policy Studies Institute (1983) points out, the denigration of women which infuses police-talk is also a devaluing of qualities associated with women that are actually required for much police work (see also Jones, 1986). Officers, therefore, avoid actions which might be taken as a sign of weakness and instead engage in aggressive behaviour:

There is a tendency in the police force at the moment to be all instant response: we all sit in the canteen and it's all instant response; you all come out rushing and you all come back, which I don't think is what policing is all about. Community beat has a different emphasis but reliefs don't appreciate that. With reliefs, rushing into situations *as a group* makes things difficult to deal with: whereas you want to act as an individual, if the situation is like getting out of hand, and you think, well what this needs is less policemen hanging around or whatever, and you've got enough common sense to realise that so you back off, you're interpreted as not getting stuck in, not being macho, which puts pressure on you. But it's not correct. They're so used to dealing with things in a confrontational way.

In the same way, categories of work which do not require resolution by coercion and which demand the service skills of negotiation, conciliation and diplomacy, are dismissed as 'grief' or 'rubbish'. Those very things which, as we saw in Chapter 3, are prominent concerns of residents: noise, pollution, stray dogs, kids playing, dumped cars and the rest, as well as 'domestic incidents', are all considered by many officers as unworthy of their attention (see also *Guardian*, letters, 28 and 30 March 1991). In part this is because officers are result-oriented in the limited sense that they want to deal with crime and achieve convictions (a crucial measure of their own success within the force), and in part because they feel they do not have the skills needed to resolve the issue (see Fielding, 1988b). The skills in question are principally verbal skills involving the ability to 'talk to people', to 'get along with the community', to 'chat about this and that', to 'talk the person down', and many officers told us that these were lacking in relief officers. Thus:

*Community beat officer interview*
Q: How can you earn the respect of the relief?
A: It can only be when they take an interest in what you're doing and come out with you. But when you tell them they are going to a meeting it frightens them to death; they won't go.

Whether officers had a skill-deficit in this respect or whether the hurried style of relief policing imposed constraints upon the use of conversational skills, officers constantly underplayed the value of talking to people ('there isn't time', 'You have to leave things when the radio goes', 'the community beats do that') and were blind to the consequences of their style of policing. Indeed, when talking about 'domestics', relief officers often phrased their actions in terms of utilizing their confrontational skills:

Domestics, my favourite subject! It can be griefy, you can go in there and it's very difficult to tell someone, say they might have been married twenty years, 'Oi, you know, what are you doing? What are you playing about at?', you know? To give them advice is quite difficult on your initial approach. You go in there, and you're going to weigh the people up, if they're going to listen to you, you can talk to them. If not, you've got to sort of say: 'OK, look. I'm the referee in this one you will now listen to me, and you'll do it this way.'

The general lack of interest in 'domestics' was confirmed to us by a former street training instructor who told us that it was impossible to instil sensitive values in many young officers. Their approach to 'domestics' was simply that they would acquire the experience of handling one situation, create a pro-forma method of dealing with it, which would then be uncritically applied to all other domestics:

> Now, dealing with a domestic situation as they sometimes call it, going to a house where domestic violence may have taken place, they want to have the experience of dealing with something like that but I don't think they go there and deal with these things really with an intention of actually sorting anything out. It's just 'Right, I've done a domestic dispute now'. I don't think they go initially with an attitude of 'There's a problem here with this family. What steps can I take to do something for the victims, the children? Can I help the woman take out an injunction against this man?.' They tend to want to get it dealt with and 'That's how I'll deal with 'em all' type of thing. Again, it's not a victim-orientated approach to dealing with anybody as far as I can see. They want to get to know the system and how they can fit into the system, and customer care is low priority to them.

At base, therefore, there is a fundamental issue of police culture. This culture is antipathetic towards the service model of policing, has little time for community policing ideals, and does not value community beat work. The overwhelming majority of officers we encountered in the Metropolitan and Avon and Somerset Police wished to pursue objectives defined as important by *them*, not those defined as important by the public. This collective sense of mission legitimated a style of policing which found its expression in action. The values espoused revolve around action rather than crime, though in the idealized world of the rank and file officer these values are often *expressed* in terms of crime or major public order confrontations. In this setting, authentic policing involves doing things to the community, not doing things for the community: real policing is concerned centrally with the imposition of control and the affirmation of police authority.

It is against this background that allegiance to a form of policing which is remote from the public and isolated has to be understood. The police as a group, as other commentators have reported (Clark, 1965; Alex, 1976; Reiner, 1978), are characterized by internal solidarity and social isolation. In part, social isolation is a by-product of identifiable features of police work: the shift system, unpredictable hours, public suspicion, fear and hostility towards authority, the need to entrench internal group solidarity, and recruitment policies which sever officers from their local communities (Miller, 1977).

But isolation is not simply a price, it is also a value. As such, it is actively sought after by relief officers, who do not disguise their wish to avoid contacts with the public which are other than transitory and superficial:

> Personally, I am not that interested in getting heavily involved in the community in any sort of formal way.

> I don't particularly wish to meet the community.

The value of isolation is that it enables officers to engage in impositional styles of control free from the contradictions that might flow from close knowledge of those policed. Treating the public as the objects of policing rather than as people in their own right both enables and legitimates an 'impersonal' style of policing that is marked by imposition and despatch.

> As a relief officer, you can get called to situations and you deal with them as you see fit, i.e. you go to a domestic disturbance, both people can be arrested for breach of the peace, if it comes to that they are arrested for breach of the peace. If I was a [CBO] I might have to go and talk to those people for the next ten years. So you're not so involved, you're there to deal with what's going on as opposed to, you've got to worry 'I've got to work this ground for that amount of time'.

> You have got to think in terms of – it's very difficult to do a job and be totally independent, unbiased, and if you don't get to know people too well you can go up to their car, you can slap a parking ticket on it, if you don't know them too well you can do them for throwing a bit of litter down in the street, whatever. If you don't know them at all they are just Joe Soap, it doesn't matter. But if you get to know them very very well as a community policeman does, it is extremely difficult to see that friend of yours who has not committed a big sin, but he has parked his car on the double yellow lines. What do you do? If you don't know him, easy.

> I think actually if you really analyse it, grief comes down to being personal. People want to discuss problems with you. It's all to do with that mentality which is we rush around and deal with

things like a Task Force and you haven't really got time to talk to people or sit down and give them a bit of sympathy. It's all tied in with rushing around and not wanting to be involved – it's probably a spin off from the isolation.

## THE OBJECTS OF POLICING

Whilst there is a well-documented police culture which predisposes the police to act in particular ways, the police also hold a set of conceptions about the public which determine how and when potential action will be operationalized. Underpinning the broad 'them' and 'us' outlook of the police, are particular typologies of the public which enable the force to refine operational strategies and target them against 'appropriate' individuals and groups. As Shearing (1981a, 1981b) points out, the way in which the police classify the public makes available to them a social theory that they can use to define situations and to construct a course of action in response.

### The decent public

In general the public are seen by the police as their allies in the fight against crime and wrongdoing. What helps provide the police with their sense of mission is the belief that they represent the views of the vast majority of the population. In this conception, the distinction between right and wrong is clear, and readily understood. This understanding of public support is based on belief, not on knowledge, but is constantly reinforced by the daily routines which involve contact only with 'the minority'. Constant contact with the minority of wrongdoers both explains for the police their cynicism ('We only see the worst of people', 'We never see the good side of society') and confirms their conviction that anyone (that is, any decent person) would share their evaluation of those they have to process. All this is to be taken for granted because the silent majority are *silent*.

> You'll find that with our job in particular you only come across a very small minority of the population. Either those that we want because they have done something wrong or those that want us for various reasons, like victims of some crime. The vast majority of the population never come into contact with the

police, maybe once or twice they get pulled up for a silly motoring offence or whatever. But most people never come into contact with the police. I would say that round here, although it doesn't look a very nice area to work, and we come across people who really are what I would call slag – they don't like us and we don't like them, because we are always being called to deal with them – but they are a very small minority. There are a lot of decent people who live here trying to get on with their lives. And they have probably been born here and brought up here, lived here all their lives. And so we as police officers tend to get a rather narrow view because we only come into contact with these certain types of people.

In [x area], the response you get down there from the public is very negative on the whole. That doesn't mean to say that the vast majority of them don't appreciate what you're doing at all, but the vast majority don't really want to be seen to be getting involved with any police officer. You get the element down there, and it's only a small element of trouble-makers and criminals, who don't like that at all and the older generation especially are scared.

The ones we meet, I wouldn't say [respond] nicely. . . . I mean, I do believe we get a lot of support, but these people never voice their opinions, probably frightened to.

This does not mean, however, that the police are willing to act on the basis of the judgement of the respectable public. On the contrary, in the police view the public's judgement cannot be relied upon. The police require from the public their tacit support but nothing else. The reason for this, as Shearing (1981b) observes, is that the public do not always respect police professionalism or acknowledge their own incompetence as lay people. Operational encounters with the public serve as a constant reminder to the police that the public do not understand what the police do, expect too much of the police, and have no knowledge of the criminal element of society which is a source of so much trouble for the force. There is no contradiction between the idealized conception of public support and the reality of less than positive encounters with the non-criminal public, because the police theorize that unqualified support would be forthcoming if only the public were better informed and more knowledgeable.

I think everyone expects too much of the police. For example, I went to a four-car road accident where the offending vehicle had crashed and the driver had run off. The vehicle was registered to somebody else and they expect you to be able to trace the driver. They think you can do all sorts of wonderful things . . . fingerprints . . . and track down the driver, but in reality you can't do that. They think you can solve a lot more crimes than you can.

Say you've been on the ground for seven hours and you've had a couple of really nasty calls, which you can have, then the last thing you need is somebody giving you a mouthful when you've done nothing except just stop them for a routine offence or check. If their opening gambit is 'Have you got nothing better to do?' or 'Shouldn't you be out catching this, that and the other?', it does put your back up a little bit. It's difficult to swallow sometimes, and that's why some members of the public think we're all nasty.

People have an inherent belief that they see a uniform and expect a solution; and when you explain that your actions can be unlawful, they don't always understand.

You tend to get that old fashioned attitude or idea, you know, that the police can do absolutely everything. There are things that they come up with like parking, and cars that are abandoned and you know, they expect the police to tow the cars away. Another thing that happens is the trouble with burglar alarms . . . if you get a burglar alarm go off, somebody goes up and checks the premises obviously, and then we get the key-holder's whereabouts, because generally they go off at odd hours of the time when nobody is there, like the thing goes off at night and we don't have any keyholder's details so then they say, 'Oh can't you do anything about it, we were told by somebody that the police will go and switch the alarm off?'. And we say 'Well we haven't got keys to go and switch it off', 'Well can't you go up there and interfere with the alarm?', that sort of thing.

I'd like to put all the anti-police people behind a riot shield at the Tottenham riots and throw burning petrol all over them. Then they'll think: 'My God! The police are marvellous.'

In the world of the rank and file officer, the public contribute little to the needs of operational policing; they do not know anything about the criminal classes, construe suspicious behaviour as unexceptionable, and are unwilling to act as informants or witnesses; they treat the police as there to do their bidding: they call the police for anything, expect an instant response, demand (not request) action, and expect the police to perform miracles; they have poor judgement and suspect motives, they invoke the authority of the police to settle old scores, they cannot distinguish police and non-police matters, and are liable 'to go over the top' if allowed to intervene themselves.

## The rough and the respectable

Since the public cannot be relied upon to assist in the definition of the police mandate or its implementation, officers are thrown back upon police culture, their sense of collective wisdom, and police professionalism. In contrast to public understandings of crime and of the police, for officers police culture is informed and knowledgeable, directed against those who represent a danger to society, forged in the crucible of operational experience, and underpinned by the highest motives. Although, as Reiner (1985, p. 94) observes, the crucial divisions made by the police do not readily fit sociological categories of class or status, police understandings of social divisions within society do reflect power structures mediated through the specific problems of police work (Reiner, 1978; Lee, 1981; Holdaway, 1983). Whilst writers have identified a complex range of police-relevant social categories, the 'fundamental division is between rough and respectable elements, those who challenge or those who accept the middle-class values of decency which most police revere' (Reiner, 1985, p. 94).

This basic division was very apparent in the way officers described the areas they policed and how they explained the differential reception they received from one area to another:

> I would say the vast majority of the public don't have a great deal of feeling of being favourable or unfavourable towards the police, and they accept that we are busy and they accept we have a difficult job to do. . . . You then have quite a large group that are very strongly behind the police, and the type of person that would say 'Would you like to come in for a cup of tea?', who

tend to be perhaps the more better off or higher in the social order, and thirdly, you have those that are against us.

It's a fairly affluent society in [this area], the people are responsive, they're thoughtful, they like the police involvement, so generally I think it's the class of people who are living here that dictates the pro-police attitude.

This fractionalization of the population was clearly seen in police understandings of people who lived in poorer quality housing, especially council estates. Whilst some police were careful to distinguish 'rough' and 'respectables' within these areas, nevertheless council estates as a whole represented for police in all three force areas the rough element of society. These were the areas, it was said, which contained the significant anti-police faction, housed the criminogenic families, and were a constant source of problems for the police:

On the estates you get more crime and domestics. Some of these are the dregs of the earth, where the council estates are.

The area is broken down into estates, residential estates and council. Council estates I would say are the brunt of our problem. Crime stems from the children who live on these estates: they grow up into adults and continue with their criminal activities.

Well obviously, like any area, you've got your bad points and your good points. You've got the estates which are generally where you get the most trouble.

As for policing problems, you've always obviously got the estates, they can be problems. It's just like a dumping ground for all the people that are not wanted, so it is always going to be a problem.

Although concern about council estates is clear in all force areas, it is black people who epitomize for the police (and for other groups in the community: Solomos, 1988, 1989) the ills of society.

**The police and black people**

Police attitudes towards black people are well documented in both the United States of America and England. In the United States, beginning with the work of Westley (1970), studies have shown that police officers hold negative, stereotyped and prejudiced attitudes towards black people (Skolnick, 1966; Bayley and Mendelsohn, 1968; Reiss, 1971; Rossi *et al.*, 1974). The British evidence is absolutely in line with these findings. Beginning with the early studies of Lambert (1970) and Cain (1973), who found a pattern of prejudice and hostility to black people in city forces, numerous research studies have uncovered a range of negative attitudes in the lower ranks of the police (Reiner, 1978, 1985; Southgate, 1982; Gordon, 1983; Holdaway, 1983; Policy Studies Institute, 1983; Fielding, 1988a; Foster, 1989; Graef, 1989; Pearson *et al.*, 1989). Our research provides striking confirmation of the continuance of these attitudes.

Although interviews with the police did not directly deal with attitudes towards black people, we found, as had Reiner (1985), that officers spontaneously advanced views about ethnic minorities. Almost one-third of Metropolitan relief officers and almost two-fifths of those in Avon and Somerset advanced negative views of black people in the course of taped interviews. There was only a handful of comparable opinions voiced by Gwent officers. The unsympathetic and derogatory views of London and Avon and Somerset officers were sometimes qualified with caveats relating to older black people, who were generally viewed as more friendly towards the police. It is important that we convey the depth of the feelings which emerged in these interviews.

In the first place black people in general but especially black youths are seen as anti-authority or, and this is much the same for most officers, anti-police. This manifests itself, according to officers, in an insolent or disrespectful attitude to the police, involving ignoring officers, making disrespectful gestures, and generally exhibiting an uncooperative attitude:

*Metropolitan relief officer*
When you walk in [to certain areas] you could try and talk to somebody. And they will suck very loudly between their teeth, which is an insult in their way of doing things. Also, you get, they don't use so much the words like 'you fucking pig' and all this business, its Yardy talk of i.e. 'you blood clot' and everything like that, or they go the other way and totally blank you out. They will not speak to you, they will not acknowledge your existence. Even if you speak to them, if they don't want to know

they will blank you out. Suck between their teeth, turn their back on you and walk off.

*Avon and Somerset community beat officer*
They carry the biggest chip on their shoulder you've ever seen: 'You only arrest them because of their colour', that's the only reason they're ever arrested or stopped, because they are black!

*Metropolitan relief officer*
I would say a lot of the younger blacks have got a big chip on their shoulder. I don't know if it's authority or not, what they're against, and if you speak to the older blacks, a lot of them have got all the time in the world for you because they respect law and order. And I was talking to a publican here and he turned round and these are his words, not mine: 'To keep a negro in order you've got to suppress him', and be that right or wrong I don't know. The younger blacks we are having problems with, the older ones are normally as good as gold.

In the second place, black people are seen to be of low intelligence, who will not listen to advice, and who act in an excitable and aggressive fashion without cause:

*Metropolitan relief officer*
The trouble, frankly, with this area is that the vast majority of black people are as thick as two short planks. They give you nothing but grief and hassle and you can't *explain* anything to them: they never see the point, even if you're trying to make it easy for them. (original emphasis)

*Gwent relief officer*
Unfortunately, it's a fact of life, members of the Afro-Caribbean nations tend to be excitable, and because of bad police press, public relations, whatever, they do tend to take the attitude they are being picked on.

*Avon and Somerset relief officer*
The majority of them just don't understand. They are of low intelligence. They've got no motivation to find a job; it's far too easy for them to go round in gangs shoplifting and things like that.

*Metropolitan relief officer*
There is high unemployment in the area so a lot of the youths,

shall we call them, hang around on the street corners, they are drinking all day, they are smoking cannabis or other drugs and they just get themselves all excited and because they are Caribbean/Jamaican their personalities – they get very excited very easily, so anything that happens they don't leave the police to get on with it, they want to know what is happening, they'd all want to try and join in and it's that type of thing that causes all the problems.

*Metropolitan relief officer*
The coloured population get very, very wound up very quickly. They're very sort of aggressive people naturally and they tend to shout. . . . And when they get upset, obviously the level goes up even more. They do tend to fling their arms around, and the situation gets out of hand.

In the third place, black people are seen to have a pathological propensity to commit crimes, especially those involving street robberies and drugs:

*Metropolitan inner-city probationary officer*
The problem is – it is very difficult to say – you can't comment on the black community without people saying you are racist. . . . I have got nothing against blacks at all. . . . Another thing here is . . . every robbery is a racial attack black against white, 80 per cent are muggers, blacks; but these statistics are just washed over. They wouldn't be publicized because it would be seen as racist – but it's a fact, and it should be attacked from that angle.

*Metropolitan community beat officer*
In the canteen, a lot of the canteen staff are black and there's jokes like between them about black people or whatever, which are all light-hearted but I don't think they actually realize that those jokes could upset people. And as for racist comments police constables are of the general belief that there is something intrinsic about black people which cause them to commit crime. They don't sit around discussing 'maybe it's the social setting they grew up in' or whatever, it's because they are black and that is the general view that is expressed.

*Avon and Somerset relief officer*
I wouldn't advise you to walk down [x] Road by yourself

because there's a chance that if there's not a police van about, you'll get mugged, because there's gangs of black kids who wait there to pick on unsuspecting people. . . . They know nothing different. Me, I've always been brought up to know the difference between right and wrong . . . maybe you do sometimes do a few things that are wrong but you know when you've done it. But the majority of the kids down there don't even know the difference. They've got their own codes of practice.

When Lord Scarman considered this question in relation to the Metropolitan Police and their role in the street disorders in Brixton in 1981, he acquitted 'senior officers of the force' of racism and located the problem of discrimination, insofar as it existed, in 'the ill-considered, immature and racially prejudiced actions of some officers in their dealings on the streets with young black people' (1981, p. 105). Ours was not a study of senior officers, and those few whom we did interview tended to express views consistent with those which confronted Lord Scarman. These officers, of course, are not generally involved in street policing, although they once were. In relation to rank and file officers we would point out that the racist sentiments we encountered were prevalent among all levels of experience: probationers, recent recruits and more experienced officers. Such attitudes can have a destructive effect upon ethnic minority people who join the police force, as the well-publicized case of Surinder Singh (a constable subjected to racist treatment by his Nottinghamshire police colleagues and discriminated against on the grounds of colour when seeking to join the detective squad) graphically shows (see Campbell, 1990). Whether such attitudes translated into discriminatory behaviour towards outsiders is something to which we now turn.

## DISCRIMINATORY BEHAVIOUR?

However shocking expressions of prejudice by police officers may be, it would be a serious mistake to assume that such prejudices necessarily lead officers to behave in discriminatory ways. It is quite possible, for example, for officers to adopt conventional police typologies about groups of people in society, called 'slag', 'toe-rags', 'scum', 'rubbish' and other epithets well known to all researchers in this area, but to carry out their operational policing duties conscientiously and without fear or favour. Establishing casual relationships on these questions is notoriously difficult and commentators have rightly warned against the danger of slipping into easy judgements and drawing unjustified inferences (see Reiner, 1985). It is important, however, to examine the question of whether the underrepresentation of NW schemes in black and working-class areas is in any way linked to their policing experiences.

The weight of research evidence, expertly reviewed by Reiner (1985, pp. 124–36), clearly establishes differential police treatment of young, economically-marginal lower-class males, especially black males. In the United States, for example, the San Diego Field Interrogation Study found that two-thirds of those stopped by the police belonged to ethnic minority groups (black or Mexican-American), a similar proportion were juveniles, and all were male (Boydstun, 1975). Research in Dallas produced comparable findings (Bogolmony, 1976), and several studies demonstrate that young, black or lower-class suspects are more likely to be arrested (Black, 1970, 1972; Sykes and Clark, 1975; Lundman et al., 1978; Lundman, 1980).

British evidence is consistent with this picture. A whole line of studies shows that young males, especially if unemployed or black, or both, are disproportionately subject to stops and stop-searches in the street by the police: Brogden, 1981; Tuck and Southgate, 1981; Field and Southgate, 1982; Willis, 1983; McConville, 1983; Policy Studies Institute, 1983; Southgate and Ekblom, 1984; Dixon et al., 1989. The pattern for arrests follows that for stops. The Home Office analysis of the 1975 Metropolitan Police statistics (Stevens and Willis, 1979), for example, found that the arrest rate for Afro-Caribbeans was higher than that for whites (and for Asians) for all offence categories. Comparable findings are reported in Field and Southgate, 1982, and Policy Studies Institute, 1983. Finally, once arrested, juveniles who are working class (Bennett, 1979; Fisher and Mawby, 1982) or black (Landau, 1981; Landau and Nathan, 1983) are more likely to be charged and prosecuted as opposed to being cautioned.

Taken together, the evidence from research justifies the conclusion of the Policy Studies Institute (1983, vol. iv, p. 166) that

It is . . . clear that the weight of police activity bears much more heavily on sections of the lower working class and others whom the police tend to lump with them than on other groups: much police activity is a way of 'dealing with' the most petty offences committed within this social milieu.

It does not follow, however, that differential treatment arises from police *discrimination*, that is, the use of police powers unjustified by legally relevant factors (Reiner, 1985, p. 129). One argument (favoured by the police) is that police attention is deserved, arising from the tendency of some individuals and groups (such as young, working-class, and black males) to over-offend. The opposing view traces differential treatment to the police tendency to stereotype people and, in consequence, to actively look for those believed to be engaged in criminal behaviour. The difficulties of establishing causal relationships on this question can be seen by looking at two studies, one in the United States of America and one in England.

In the United States, the observational study of Black and Reiss (Black, 1970, 1972), concluded that the disproportionate rate of black arrests was not a product of discriminatory treatment but due to the interactional relationship between the police and citizen in which black people more frequently displayed disrespect for the police. Whilst this line of analysis finds support in other research, later research found that in about half of all cases, disrespect could have been a *product* of the behaviour of the police themselves (Sykes *et al.*, 1976; and see Smith and Visher, 1981). A similar problem surrounds the leading British study. The Policy Studies Institute in seeking to explain negative assessments of the police made by Afro-Caribbeans concluded that

> the hostility of West Indians (and young West Indians in particular) to the police cannot be explained by the way in which they themselves were treated by the police in specific instances, though it may be explained, at least in part, by the large *number* of contacts they have had and by the very high *proportion* of contacts in which they were being treated as offenders or suspects rather than getting help or advice.
>
> (1983, vol. iv, p. 333)

This, as Lea (1986) points out, is contradictory. Police behaviour is said not to have contributed to hostile opinions about the force but, as the Policy Studies Institute shows, negative opinion increases with the frequency of being stopped, and police stops are not justified by legally relevant criteria. As the Policy Studies Institute report shows elsewhere, the question of what their legal powers may be 'does not enter into [police] decision-making except in the case of rare individuals' (p. 233). Rather, the police

> strongly tend to choose young males, especially young black males. Other groups that they tend to single out are people who look scruffy or poor ('slag'), people who have long hair or unconventional dress . . . and homosexuals.

> (ibid.)

The links in the chain of influences and causation are thus unclear and there is little hope of settling this question satisfactorily. None the less, the point is important and our research has thrown up material which bears on the issue. These findings, we wish to emphasize, are by no means conclusive but are in line with the findings of Foster (1989) in her study of Metropolitan Police officers and they support the conclusion of careful reviews of the research (Reiner, 1985; Brogden et al., 1988) that differential treatment is *in part* a product of discriminatory treatment by the police. Our study discloses three types of evidence suggestive of police discrimination: (i) public experiences and perceptions of policing; (ii) concerns expressed by officers about the attitudes and behaviour of their colleagues; and (iii) self-reported discriminatory behaviour by officers. We shall say a little about each in turn.

## Public experiences and perceptions of policing

One of the striking findings of our research is the disjuncture between public perceptions of the police in the Metropolitan and Avon and Somerset inner-city areas and those of residents elsewhere. In the inner-city areas of London and Bristol, residents were much more sharply critical of the police and spontaneously accused the police of discriminatory behaviour, especially towards black people, as Table 6.1 shows.

*Table 6.1* Spontaneous accusations of local police discrimination against black people, inner-city London and Bristol

|  | No. of inner-city residents interviewed | Respondents alleging police racism, no. and % | |
|---|---|---|---|
| London | 53 | 18 | 34.0 |
| Bristol | 18 | 7 | 38.9 |

In addition to those listed in Table 6.1, another group of residents (10 per cent in each city) specifically called for the recruitment into the police of more black officers, and yet others were critical of insensitive or heavy-handed policing without explicitly alleging that there was a problem of racism within the police. Whilst research shows that black people, especially young black people, are more hostile to the police than other groups (Policy Studies Institute, 1983), our findings show that serious criticism is also a characteristic of white residents, male and female and of all ages. These criticisms are the more persuasive because the views of residents do not amount to an outright rejection of the value of policing; indeed, support for law and order was almost universal. Rather, public attitudes were a dialogue with the type of policing perceived to be current, and criticisms were directed to changing the policing style, not to removing the police from the community.

In London, it was common for inner-city residents to depict the police as 'racist' and to call for a very substantial reorganization of the force so that it more nearly reflected the racial composition of the community. Complaints related to 'harassment' of black people, unjustified stopping, searching and arresting, and, much less frequently, brutality towards black people. Overlaying all of these comments was a persistent complaint about the 'attitude' of officers. Our findings are directly in line with those of Foster (1989) in her observational study of two London police stations. In one, Foster found a 'cowboy' style of policing, marked by macho and aggressive behaviours through which young officers overcompensated for an inability to deal with people of their own age. These officers exhibited a desire for confrontation and 'winding people up' in order to create more explosive situations. She found, for example, officers acting in an aggressive and sarcastic manner, hoping that those stopped 'would rise to the bait' (1989, p. 133), the use of abusive (including racist) language towards citizens, and conduct specifically designed to provoke a hostile reaction and thus to legitimate an aggressive response. Our research supports this line of analysis, with persistent complaints volunteered by residents about the aggressive, racist and hostile manner of Metropolitan Police officers. The following quotations from white residents in London illustrate these points:

There should be less harassment especially on black people

because I've been at scenes where black people are arrested. They are getting caught for no apparent reason.

They are always very pleasant to me which you would expect them to be to a doctor and someone from this neighbourhood. Very pleasant. I think they probably have an extremely difficult job. . . . The police have always been nice to me. On the other hand I have seen them stopping coloured youths in the street sometimes and as I've walked past, heard them talking to them. I certainly didn't like the way they were talking to them at all. The tone they were using was a sort of harassing tone. Though they certainly wouldn't use it on someone like me, I don't think police ought to talk like that.

I'm not satisfied with the attitude of the police force in general to racial problems. They've tried to change it, bring in coloured policemen sort of thing, but it's a surface thing. It's basically the attitude of white policemen to coloured people is basically appalling actually, so how you change that, it's ingrained, I don't quite know what the answer is. This is at the root of a lot of problems. Sensitive is the answer. That's not being very specific but a sensitive, thoughtful approach to people. If people see that the police are being sensitive they will get more respect. When the police become bullies they lose all the respect they have. Needless violence to coloured people makes the situation worse.

The police are obviously not doing a good job. They could stop harassing people for driving nice cars, they could stop harassing people because of the way they dress, without due reason. I know loads of guys that because of the car they are driving get constantly stopped. Police hassle them with 'What do you expect? It's a BMW and you are black', that sort of thing.

Parallel sentiments were expressed by inner-city residents in Bristol, who perceived the police as being antagonistic and unfair towards local black people, as well, occasionally, to other groups low in the hierarchy of social power. The following quotes from white residents in inner-city Bristol demonstrate these concerns:

There does seem to be a scale of attention or trust they give to people and black people do seem to be at the bottom of the scale. They'll hassle them first, then round this area you've got squatters and punks and they're next on the scale then it goes up to the old age pensioners who don't get hassled. The stupid thing is most of the muggings are caused by a white middle class gang, though they don't operate much any more but they wouldn't get as much hassle as a black kid.

Q: Are you satisfied with your local police?

A: Yes, it looks as though they're trying but they've got a problem in Bristol. They're racist, they don't like black people. A friend of ours is a teacher and some cops swore at her, just because she's black. A black neighbour was driving his Mum's white GTI convertible and he stopped at a chip shop and the police asked him to stop but he didn't and they got the address from the computer and they accused him of stealing the car. He's not allowed to drive a smart car because he's black. The crime rate is quite high here but it's probably not the blacks' fault. I know if I'm attacked in the streets round here and I shout everyone will come out; that doesn't happen in Redland and Clifton. If our next door neighbours who are Jamaican hear anything they'll call the cops.

I suppose it has to start with the training, training for the kind of areas they are going to go into and perhaps a bit more sensitivity. Better handling of situations; sometimes they probably aggravate the situation by insensitive handling. Perhaps the way they speak to people. Like talking rudely, I have seen them pull up a black guy and say 'Where are you going boy?', I just feel that he is a grown man and there is no need to speak to him like that. If he was white, would they have done that or would they have said 'Excuse me sir, where are you going? Can you help us with our questioning?', which might have saved a lot of aggro had they approached the black guy in the same way. He might have said 'I am going to so and so and would be quite happy to help you'.

In both London and Bristol, allegations of physical brutality, assaults and the like by the police were confined to a few isolated instances. The complaints related much more, as these illustrations make clear, to racist attitudes, 'harassment' or 'hassling' of a non-specific character, and the disproportionate use of stop and arrest powers. This impression was, in a few instances, reinforced by the way in which officers responded to incidents in which the resident had been victimized. Residents reported that the police were quick to assume that the offender was black and sometimes transmitted their prejudices in clear ways, as in the following examples:

> It would help if the police had a more relaxed attitude when they come [to the estate], because I've heard them say 'It's another bloody black bastard anyway probably', which doesn't help.

> When we were burgled, either you get someone who comes in, like the policeman who came to us, and says 'Yeah, well, this was obviously done by a coon!' I thought, 'That's very constructive', especially as I knew who it was done by and who is actually white. I can remember I employed a nanny who was black, and after two months she disappeared in the middle of the night, and she left all her clothes here. Then the next day, she broke in through the French windows, went up to her bedroom, packed all her clothes in a bag, and left. Didn't take anything else, but I reported it because I wanted to get the windows mended on the insurance. It was as simple as that. She *was* wonderful with the children, but the thing is that she did have a typical W. Indian walkabout mentality; if she said she was going out for one and a half hours, you were quite likely to see her four days later. She had no sense of time, or the work ethic in her, in the way that is normally instilled in people. . . . Anyway, she disappeared, and when this happend, when I reported it, the policeman said 'Right, I'm going round. Know where she lives?' I gave him the address, and when he came round again, just to get his report all sorted out, he said 'Cor, I tell you what. I went round there and scared the shit out of her. She won't do that to anybody again.' So I said, 'Oh, is she all right?', 'cos she was actually lovely with the children. He said, 'You're fucking mad employing a black girl to look after your kids. I mean, anything could've happened.' And I thought 'Fine . . . thanks a lot . . . I won't do it again!'

**Concerns expressed by officers about their colleagues**

In line with other observational research, we overheard racist comments and 'jokes' in police canteens in which black people were referred to as 'coons', 'niggers', 'spades', 'spooks', 'shadows' and other derogatory epithets. Moreover, as with other researchers, we did not encounter any example of an officer openly objecting to what was said (see for example Policy Studies Institute, 1983, vol. 4, p. 120). In private, however, a few officers took the opportunity to distance themselves from the attitudes and behaviour of their colleagues. Thus whilst some senior officers took the line, so devastatingly criticized by Hall (1979), that racism in the police was no more than a reflection of general societal prejudice, others were far less complacent, as the following example from London shows:

> I think for many [officers] it takes an awful long time to get through to them, if we ever do get through to them. I find the attitude of certain police officers distresses me greatly towards the public, in their conversations with people, attitude towards people. There are certain police officers who in their own esteem put themselves above the community and see the public as an annoyance to them in their working life. Senior management in the police force will always say 'Oh that's not the case. There are many officers who are doing a very good job in the community.' That is true, but in my experience they tend to be the odd individuals who've seen the light, so to speak, and who do realise that they work for the people of this country and that is who they owe their allegiance to. I still see a lot of police officers, and to me it's the majority, who see that their responsibility is first and foremost is to the Metropolitan Police and not the people of England.

A few rank and file officers were also critical of some of their colleagues, although they evidenced no concern to avoid working with them and showed no interest in making a complaint about their attitudes or behaviour (on which, see Chapter 7). One London officer, who reported that he had recently been granted his ideal posting to community beat work, went to considerable efforts to tell us the extent of the problem of police culture and the mechanisms by which it finds expression in dealings with the public. Although other officers talked of colleagues 'going over the top', 'not acting in a professional manner', 'coming on strong' and other euphemistic expressions, we reproduce below an extensive extract from this officer in order to demonstrate how causal relationships may be constituted:

Q: Could you describe to me what it was like working as a relief officer?

A: The expectations I had have not been fulfilled; they have not been matched up with the experience. That isn't the job itself but the people in the job you have to work with: the level of courtesy current amongst officers leaves something to be desired; the basic attitudes and values of the established police constable leaves something to be desired. This feeling about the attitudes of officers from my probationary period is not just myself but was shared by other probationary officers as well.

Q: What sorts of attitude did you encounter which you didn't like among the relief officers?

A: The basic lack of intellectual interest is very prevalent, plus subtle racism and sexism.

Q: How did these attitudes surface?

A: Say in the canteen, general chit chat, when you are out; not particularly overt but subtle. When they stop you, they are more aggressive and less sympathetic than they would be to someone else who was not black.

Q: If they are more aggressive and if racism is subtle, would it be picked up by the person being spoken to?

A: Yes. It would be picked up on the way that the person showed an immediate dislike to him. If they just arrested someone then he'd set about them: rather than saying, even if this person has done something really obnoxious like robbed some old lady, they'd say, rather than just say 'You've just mugged an old man' or whatever, they'd say 'You black shit' which really isn't relevant and is bound to upset and antagonise people.

Q: Did you find that aggressive attitudes caused the person spoken to to be aggressive back to the officers?

A: Yes, yes. I found that *generally* with policemen. Where a more easy going approach would be more appropriate they tend to expect, they tend to expect too much submissiveness from people when they are dealing with them. And there is no reason why people should be submissive, especially if they are treated in an aggressive way, especially young people. They antagonise people and then wind them up and end up arresting them for something they wouldn't have arrested them [for] if the attitude of the officer had been correct.

I've been out with officers who I think their behaviour and their way of dealing with people is better than mine and I'd like to emulate them – speaking to people, getting along with them, having the gift of the gab sort of thing. But as a rule, I don't enjoy going out with officers because their attitude and values conflict with mine and the way they talk to people: it's like I find it embarrassing. Like, if you stop someone in a car that is not wearing their seatbelt, I'd point out to them, and if at the end of the day they won't accept they've got to put their seatbelt on I'd report them, not just for their attitude. But other PCs they start off by leaning in the car window and say; 'Does it work?' and the person doesn't know *what* they are talking about; 'Does it work?' and the person will say 'Sorry?' and then they go 'Your seatbelt, does it work?'. Well I think 'Oh God let's get out of here, it's so embarrassing' and that's just like typical of, well, *all* of them.

Q: How do people react to this sort of treatment?

A: Obviously they, . . . if they don't do anything, they are obviously embittered by the form of address so they just button their lip and take it out on the next policeman; often people like young people and some young black people who haven't got much respect for the police as a rule, quite rightly in some instances, he doesn't have to take that sort of thing, he won't be rude but will answer back and that just leads to a stepping up of the PC's level of aggression and it turns nasty and he ends up reporting him for something he wouldn't have reported him for. Or it turns into a bigger issue like, well the first person really gets out of his tree and gets arrested for breach of the peace which would never have happened if it wasn't for the copper's attitude in the first place in being aggressive with them. (original emphasis)

We see here, supporting Foster's (1989) research findings, how prejudice may be easily communicated to the citizen and lead to spiralling hostility, which ultimately results in official action unrelated to the reason for the initial intervention. It is not even necessary to look for overt acts of aggression or manifest hostility on the part of the police, although these are also reported in stark form (for examples see the *Guardian*, 26 July 1990, p. 5, reporting an out of court settlement by the Metropolitan Police for £20,000 arising out of complaints by four young black men against the police for abuse and assault; and the *Guardian*, 24 November 1990, reporting the High Court action by the black boxer Maurice Hope for false arrest and wrongful imprisonment in which the Metropolitan Police paid £50,000 damages in settlement of the claim without prejudice to the issue of liability). Instead, there is a continuum of fear and violence, so that prejudice may be conveyed by manner, demeanour, inflexion or tone, each powerful enough to elicit negative responses which, to a less astute observer, would mistakenly be thought of as uninvited and unprovoked. In this way, violence is expressed in terms of the fear used by state officials to regulate and discipline sections of the community (Poulantzas, 1969, pp. 77–8) thought to have a pathological tendency to engage in 'trouble'.

## Self-reported discriminatory behaviour

Whatever the precise causal links, it is abundantly clear that police–community relations in the inner-city areas of London and Bristol are poor. And the predictable consequence of this set of relationships is that the behaviour of each side will be affected when any encounter actually occurs. Not only this, the perceptions held by each side affect when and where encounters are likely to take place. All this emerged consistently in the way officers described their work practices in interviews with us.

In the first place, since the nature of police–community relations largely reflected police typologies of the population, pro-active police behaviour heavily focused upon the poorer sections of the community. 'Suspicion', therefore, could be satisfied in the police view by membership of a class of people thought to be criminogenic:

*Avon and Somerset officer*
If I see a man in a suit walking around an affluent area, I wouldn't think a lot about it. However, if I saw a coloured person walking around [in x] – which is a well-to-do area, I would be very suspicious, because it would strike me as out of place because there's not a lot of coloured people living up

there. . . . In my experience, it's the people from St Paul's and the housing estates that are going round doing things.

Moreover, this can in the eyes of the police justify further action even where the encounter is initially 'unproductive', as in the following example. Here, an officer from Avon and Somerset described how a car had been stopped 'on instinct', the names of the occupants had come back as 'no trace' on the computer, and the occupants had been co-operative:

Now they were quite happy about giving their details. That started the alarm bells. And in the end, short of having anything else, *they looked a little bit scruffy*, so they were nicked. It was a bit of a barbed wire act, [laughs] bending the rules to bring them in. (emphasis added)

It is clear, therefore, that police understandings of the community routinely affect pro-active police work (and, indeed, how they choose to respond to citizen-initiated complaints). It is important to realize that encounters are not simply a function of offending behaviour by the citizen but are created by the operationalization of police stereotypes. It is also clear that the views about the community held by some officers have a major influence upon how officers interact with the public. It requires a considerable exercise of restraint for an officer to act fairly and dispassionately in dealing with someone who is felt to be 'slag'. Yet some observational police studies report that some officers who privately express racist views can enjoy friendly relations on the street with black people (for example Black and Reiss, 1967; Policy Studies Institute, 1983). In our study, however, some officers were unable to disguise their true feelings, as the following Avon and Somerset officer demonstrates:

I would say that 80–90 per cent of the people in [the inner city] are bloody excellent people, really nice. The rest are the dregs of the earth really. Not because of their colour, because I got nothing against their colour at all, though you do tend to develop the [simulates a furtive, muttering sound] 'Black bastard!', but that's just an expression, nothing against their colour at all.

Moreover, the lack of co-operativeness or overt hostility towards the police displayed by some groups can result in officers adjusting their behaviour to suit the occasion. As a Metropolitan relief officer told us, the 'whole job is done on the "attitude test": basically you react to how people react to you'. But this 'reaction' can be *anticipatory* rather than reactive, as a Gwent officer explained in his approach to council estates:

> Simply because the majority – I won't say everybody – do tend to be anti-police, you tend to go in with a different attitude. You wouldn't go in tending to be polite, simply because they wouldn't understand what politeness is. These type of people always think they are missing out on something. A lot of this type of people tend to be unemployed and have no intentions of going back to work whatsoever. They've got no regard for cleanliness: you go into these areas, it's filthy, disgusting, their houses smell, they don't clean up, they don't wash their kids; so what chance has law and order got?

A consequence of this kind of attitude, however, is that many police officers consider that certain areas of the city are not suitable for community policing precepts. This is evidenced by the attitude of community beat officers who often view council estates and areas populated by ethnic minority groups as inappropriate for neigh-bourhood watch schemes. This view may be founded in an unsuccessful attempt to establish a scheme or it may arise directly from general prejudice, as the following responses from London community beat officers show:

> When I started out I used to walk the estate area mainly, all the time, but now I find that because it's a council area, a lot of properties and that, and because I walk on my own, I find that there are some times when I don't go down there as much as what I really should. I find that it's, after a while, when you're dealing with people and you get this negative attitude all the time, it actually rubs off on yourself, and you come to the stage of thinking well, if they don't care about things, why should I care? Especially when you've tried setting up advice centres down there, something new, tried distributing leaflets to every house down there.

> So far as neighbourhood watch is concerned, in [x Road] forget it. It's no point. Having said that, I haven't actually been round there, knocked on the doors, but I would think most of them wouldn't want to know.

In the black sections of the inner-city areas of London and Bristol (for discussion of Toxteth in Liverpool, see Law and Henfry, 1981; Scraton, 1982; and for Chapeltown, Leeds, see Rose, 1991) police policies continue to be dominated by negative historical encounters and police conceptualizations of the population as aggressive and violent. Most intensely in Bristol, where officers spoke of the daily risk of being 'bricked and bottled', of menacing crowds gathering at any incident, and of the intimidation of residents by 'criminals', officers rejected the possibility of utilizing community policing precepts. The concern for personal safety and minimizing the chances of street incidents escalating into public disorder or riots, dictated that CBOs were 'doubled-up', that suspected offenders were removed from the street 'with dispatch', and that pro-active raids were carried out with 'numerical superiority'. The resulting distrust and impositional style of policing came in for severe criticism from one officer who told us that the police did not know the community and had never offered residents community policing ideals. Wherever the truth lies here, no officer claimed that this part of the city enjoyed a policing system based upon positive interactions with citizens, and almost every officer located the problem in the attitudes and behaviour of residents and not in the attitudes and behaviour of the police.

The result inevitably is that whole areas of the community are written off by the police. The ideals of community policing find life only in the 'middle-class', 'posh' and 'propertied' areas which are continually celebrated by rank and file officers. Other areas, and classically this means large parts of council estates and the black community, lose out by default or are overtly discarded as outside the boundary of acceptable society. The following exchange with an Avon and Somerset officer typifies a very strong strand of operational policing policy:

Q: Could neighbourhood watch be set up in [a named 'sensitive' area of the city]?
A: The problem down there is that the majority of the time you're dealing with the scum. They are the scum down there.

Similarly, when we went out on the beat with one CBO in London, it became obvious that he avoided an estate that fell within his beat area. When we asked him about this estate, he said,

I don't often walk through there, I must be honest. I have got so much more to do, I don't feel it's my responsibility. The estate is full of 'scrotes' and 'shitbags' – not just any youngster who's a bad person . . . but squatters, illegal tenants and so on.

## CONCLUSION

Both policing resources and policing ideologies are dominated by a culture which finds clearest expression in the views of relief officers. This culture is essentially aggressive and action-centred, and stands in opposition to the ideals of community beat work. Community beat officers and the work they carry out are not viewed positively by relief officers in the Metropolitan and Avon and Somerset forces, and are given value only insofar as they are functional to the needs of relief. The ideologies of action, crime and aggression lead officers to devalue those matters, such as nuisance incidents and 'domestics', which are prominent concerns of the residents.

These practices are sustained by the intense solidarity of internal occupational culture and work patterns, but are also pursued as a desirable *objective*. Isolation is deliberately cultivated by officers who fear that extended community relations would complicate and confuse their mandate, and threaten the impositional style of policing which is thought to be necessary and appropriate.

This style of policing is not, however, universalized. The police have little to do with large sections of society. When contact occurs with these groups, it is non-confrontational and public trust and confidence in the police is assumed by officers. Even if citizens appear on occasion to be ungrateful or critical of police action, none the less officers are comforted by the sense of support which these communities generate.

The weight of policing falls instead upon narrow bands of society, principally council estates and black areas of the community. The differential policing treatment meted out to these sectors of society was all too apparent to residents, and acknowledged by many officers as institutional responses to 'problem' areas. Whilst causal relationships are hard to establish, the evidence shows clearly that at least some of the differential treatment is *directly* attributable to discriminatory policing. Police do not simply respond to hostile or uncooperative behaviour from ethnic minorities – although they may receive plenty of this; instead, prejudicial attitudes, strongly reinforced by occupational culture, inform the way in which the police respond to incidents involving black people.

# Chapter 7

# Institutional dynamics of police culture

Understanding police occupational culture – a white, male, action-centred sense of mission, underpinned by substantial internal solidarity and the stereotyping of individuals and groups who are 'outsiders' – is central to the debates about the problems of law enforcement in England and Wales today. The gulf between what the public want of the police and what the police actually deliver, especially in inner-city areas, cannot be explained by a failure of resources. Instead, a significant reason for both the method of policing and its temper is the culture of front-line officers, whose lack of sympathy with service policing and the rhetoric of community policy and neighbourhood watch is only too well reflected in official force policies. For officers at the sharp end of policing, community beat work is a sop to liberal society which, if it is to be undertaken at all, is a minority pursuit of misfits, or of officers approaching retirement. Core policing for them is confrontational and impositional in nature and directed against those considered to be outcasts or on the margins of society. How this culture should be understood is, then, a centrally important question and has been a matter of fierce debate.

The nature of our research, limited by the willingness of officers to reveal fully their own working philosophies, does not allow a complete answer to this debate. None the less, our research provides important data on system-wide institutional features of police culture. Our research casts grave doubt upon explanations framed in terms of individual pathology and shows how police values and ideologies are an inscribed feature of the police organization, embedded in situational working practices, and central to understanding external and internal control systems. Police culture is not monolithic and variations are discernible both from force to force and within individual forces, but the communalities that are central to our discussion are discernible in weaker or more power- ful forms in each of the forces studied. Before looking at our own data, we wish to say a little about arguments directed to explaining discriminatory actions of the police in terms of prejudiced officers.

Until relatively recently, it has been common to present the police as engaging in behaviours which are directly intended, so that the explanation for actions is located in the motivations of individual officers. This explanation has been fostered by the police themselves, who describe internal police disciplinary sys- tems as concerned with rooting out wayward officers, 'bad apples' who give the force an undeservedly bad reputation. This provides the groundwork for the argument that the police, along with other public agencies, should be expected to 'be landed with their "fair share" of prejudiced individuals' which is an inevitable result of the make-up of society as a whole and 'not something for which the police as such can be held responsible' (Lea, 1986, p. 150. See also Taylor, 1983). In these accounts it is never made clear whether 'aberrant' individuals should be eradicated simply because their presence within the police brings other officers (undeservedly) into disrepute or because of a risk that they may contaminate the 'rest of the barrel'. In any event the implicit assumption that there is nothing to say about police racism apart from what might be said about general societal racism is, as we shall see, mistaken. More- over, and insofar as this kind of argument is relied upon by the police themselves, as Hall has observed, chief constables would not state so readily the equally valid proposition that the police force must also contain its fair share of criminals (Hall, 1979, p. 13).

An enhanced version of the 'bad apple' argument traces the problem to the kinds of people who are recruited into the police. On this view, in the words of Colman and Gorman (1982) 'the police force attracts conservative and authoritarian personalities' and, whilst basic training has a temporary liberalizing effect, 'continued police service results in illiberal/intolerant attitudes' towards black people. At an empirical level, other research both in England (Cochrane and Butler, 1980; Butler, 1982) and in North America (McNamara, 1967; Bayley and Mendelsohn, 1968; Bent, 1974) suggests instead that the typical officer is no more authorit- arian in outlook than the typical citizen. Others point out that we 'cannot even be sure there is such a thing as a police personality, however loosely we define it' (More, 1976, p. 125). Even if this cannot yet be given 'sideshow status' (Fielding, 1988b, p. 5), the balance of the evidence determines that it is 'still necessary to be agnostic' (Reiner, 1985, p. 102), and that attention is more profitably focused upon the work demanded of the police and its institutional placing. It is to that institutional placing that we first turn.

## INSTITUTIONAL TENDENCIES TOWARDS A COMMON CULTURE

Police occupational culture is underpinned by a network of codes which set standards of thought and behaviour in carrying out the official police function. Whilst much policing is carried out by lone officers with substantial operational autonomy, many critical interactions with citizens involve officers acting in combination. In these encounters, situational features demand substantial agreement among officers as to what constitutes 'appropriate' policing responses both at the time of the encounter and afterwards in official accounts which have to be created, filed and authenticated. Since the presence of some 'unknown' officers can unsettle a group and inhibit common action, an important tendency in policing is 'knowing' your colleagues and socializing newcomers into prevailing norms of behaviour.

As in all forms of socialization, police demands to conform are not wholly successful. Thus, for example, in one study of recruits, 22 per cent had left the force within the first two years (Fielding, 1988b). Moreover, some individuals have the capacity to resist incorporation into a culture with which they disagree and have, for the most part, the opportunity to avoid forms of policing which involve group action by, for example, becoming community beat officers. For these and other reasons, then, the norms and values of police subculture are continually negotiated in dealing with members of the public. None the less, as we shall see, the structural dynamics of the policing organization strongly favour a common culture and the removal or 'management' of antipathetic elements.

It is important to emphasize at this point that whilst police occupational culture has its own momentum it is not autonomous in the sense of being outside the wider structures of society. On the contrary, police culture replicates these wider structures only too well. Those against whom police power is consistently deployed – the 'roughs', 'scum' and other categories referred to by Cray (1972) as 'police property' – are initially identified and constituted by the values and practices of the wider society which hands on to the police the management of 'social problems'. As Reiner put the point in relation to racism,

> The crucial source of police prejudice is societal racism which places ethnic minorities disproportionately in those strata and situations from which the police derive their 'property'. This structual feature of police ethnic minority relations bolsters any prior prejudice police officers have.
>
> (1985, pp. 102–3)

But, as the Institute of Race Relations pointed out as far back as 1979, even if 'popular morality come to define black people out of society, as an "alien wedge" or as "swamping" British culture . . . the police no longer just reflect or reinforce that morality: they recreate it. . . . Deriving their sanction from popular morality they are now become the arbiters of that morality' (Institute of Race Relations, 1979, p. 1). And the grammar of police occupational culture and its insidious nature are intimately related to the internal structure of the police, its patterns of organization, its division of labour, and the dynamics of group behaviour. It is to these internal relations that we now turn.

A core issue in understanding how occupational culture is kept in place within the police is the centrality of the relief group. Relief officers constitute over eight out of every ten police constables. These officers are assigned to distinct groups whose members work as a unit, share the same shifts, operate together when collective action or 'urgent assistance' demands, and from whose members smaller patrol groups are constituted. The group is a 'cohesive social unit' (Punch, 1979, p. 16) whose members see themselves as having to deal with the unpleasant social situations for which they receive no thanks from the public and no recognition from their superiors. Internal solidarity is thus to some extent a response to two seemingly contradictory features group members identify as distinguishing their work: its low status within the policing organization and its core value. Relief officers, who themselves stigmatize community beat work as not involving 'real' policing, feel strongly that their job is heavily undervalued within the force. In this view, working on relief is not simply a low status position but is 'the pits'. Relief is considered, therefore, as a place to which people are consigned, the bottom of the organization, the end of the line, as these relief officers make clear:

> It's obviously considered that relief PCs are considered the bottom of the pile. . . . You feel it sometimes in the general attitude. Just by saying that – 'I see you have got six years' service, why are you still on relief?' Just to say you should be moving on now with your service.

> I think the relief officers tend to be looked at as the bottom of the ladder really. You often hear that people get disciplined – they are sent back to relief as if working relief is a punishment and not something that people would enjoy – you often hear that someone who maybe is in the CID and gets disciplined, and gets sent back to uniform on relief and that's classified as a punishment. It just goes to show that they treat relief as being bottom of the ladder and that's where everybody who is going nowhere – that's where they are going to send them.

> We've probably got a standing slightly above a cadet and slightly below a police dog!

These evaluations of the relief are much easier to cope with because officers strongly feel that these are misjudgements. In their view, the relief is the backbone of all policing, the first at scenes of crime, responsive to any incident, ever ready and ever available. In this understanding, relief officers are the essential service deliverers who collectively represent 'the thin blue line':

> Reliefing is where the work's done a lot of the time. Reliefing is the soldiering, the foot-slogging on the street.

> If anyone does anything wrong in another [department] they always get kicked back to relief, so it always makes it sound as if people on relief are the worst. Whereas in fact the majority of police officers are relief officers and without them the system would fall to pieces.

These pressures towards internal solidarity are enhanced by the functional value of group cohesiveness. Officers are sometimes placed in positions of possible danger and may have to rely upon their colleagues to save them. Indeed, they need to know in advance that such assistance will be forthcoming, and this can only be so where officers share a common bond of trust and understanding. And on a more mundane level, the 'thankless' task of policing the public and being continually called upon to resolve situations where civilians 'have abdicated any personal responsibility to act' (Lee, 1981, p. 50) is eased, if not made possible, by the mutual support and comfort which a cohesive social unit provides:

> You can feel grieved, you can feel upset, angry or just plain hurt, and you can come back to the nick feeling in any of those ways, and within five or ten minutes back in the company of the relief, you're well on the way to forgetting it, because they help you through it. They'll either take the mickey out of you or there's banter or there's sympathy, or there's just plain 'look, y'know, it was a bad incident. For Christ's sake, get over it.' So that's why it's important that everybody gets on, you have to be able to rely on every person on that relief 100 per cent, because the day you might need it then when they come running you want every single one of them to break their necks to get to you. You can't afford somebody saying 'oh, I don't feel like it' or 'I had a row with him yesterday'. You can't have that. It's gotta be 100 per cent commitment to each other all the time.

But behind assertions of the value of group solidarity lies a less acceptable reality, as many officers were keen to make clear. The process of socializing newcomers into existing group norms has its origins in police training school. We found little evidence that training school was effective in instilling into new recruits attitudes and perspectives associated with community policing ideals. Attempts to improve training programmes, following the criticisms of Lord Scarman (1981), through the introduction of 'human awareness training' and 'policing skills' initiatives were not viewed positively by officers to whom we spoke. Probationers of only a few months' standing told us that they could remember little or nothing of these 'social skills' aspects of training, that they represented an insignificant part of training and that 'everyone understood you just had to sit through a morning or two of that stuff'. For some, the training had been carried out in a perfunctory manner by people who had no belief in what they were doing:

> I found the people who were teaching about racism were ignorant about the subject anyway. Rather than promoting sympathy or understanding towards other races and culture,

they actually made derogatory comments about them. As an example of their ignorance, they were giving us a lecture on different religions and the particular member of staff who was doing it, didn't know the first thing about Hinduism or Buddhism or the Sikh religion or any other religion which he was giving the lecture on. He was making statements which were in fact wrong and as an example I can remember he started the topic on Hinduism, his first comment, as an opener was 'Hindus are the most bigoted group I've ever known' which I didn't think was going to promote understanding and empathy toward this particular group.

For officers in general, training school represented 'a perfect world' which could not replicate 'the real world out there'. Whatever it tried to accomplish, therefore, always evaporated in the face of experience and the influence of officers who already had access to the insights of real policing. Training school did, however, communicate one important message to cadets, as Fielding points out:

> Novices are here for the first time in continuous contact with the police, many of whom have greater experience, but also with many of their peers as well. The latter enable a rehearsal of how occupational culture can nurture and protect its members, with exam-swotting syndicates, a social life involving those in the same groups and some of the forms of collaboration and collusion that any body of students use to survive the student role.
>
> (1988b, p. 54)

But socialization finds its fullest expression in the group setting of the relief and it commences upon induction. The initiate is made fully aware of the lowly status of the probationer and of the importance of acquiescence in group norms. The new recruit 'is continually on trial' (Fielding, 1988b, p. 65), and is *made* to feel continuously on trial with the recruit's responses to the induction process monitored and scrutinized at every moment. In one form or other, the process involves undermining the self-esteem of recruits, increasing their sense of dependency, and throwing them back upon the group:

> When you join you are a probationer and that's looked down on. I thought this was odd because whenever you join any other job, people are generally good towards you and want to help

you but within the [police] there's no need for that because PCs aren't going to get any more respect from their other colleagues and they look at probationers to take the butt of their jokes, do their crappy jobs or whatever, make the tea. It's like institutionalized being rude to people and that manifests itself in say the way the sergeant will speak to you – it wouldn't be the way he'd speak to one of the other sergeants or his inspector; not merely the words he'd use but the lack of respect that he's shown you.

(officer just out of probation)

As Stoddard (1968) shows, 'the breakdown of each new recruit's morale is an important step in gaining [the recruit's] acceptance of the "code"' which binds the group together. Some of the strategies employed to test the resolve of recruits and to assert the primacy of group norms seem petty considered in isolation and are often so described by officers when they seek to convey the effectiveness of the process. Talking about the strategies, many officers told us, could not capture the insidious and powerful nature of the group's will imposed upon the recruit. A recurrent feature of these accounts (as the following passage in which a woman officer explains the sexist approach of the group), is the unspoken force of group norms and the almost mystic way in which they command allegiance and deny contradiction:

I don't think the relief like women in the job as a group. Yet on their own, I think they are quite keen to have them there, if you know what I mean. Because I find PCs or people in the police very eager to agree with whoever has the loudest mouth in the canteen, because again they don't want to be shoved out of the group. There might be someone on the relief who's having a little bit of a difficult time, maybe he didn't deal with an incident that the rest of the relief thought he should have gone and dealt with. There may have been a perfectly good reason why the person didn't deal with it, and everyone thinks they're lazy. It's almost like a boarding school, you've got like the prefects if you like, and it goes down in stages and you've got the first year pupils, and if you don't look as if you are keen and interested, and [don't] really want to get on and take any arrest that comes your way and deal with any paperwork, then they won't accept you. But then again, you can do absolutely bugger all but have the personality that agrees with the group that is in charge of that relief if you like and you will get on. People who don't do any work at all, hardly ever do any work at all right from the beginning. Yet because of their personality, and they're good fun to be with and they are a good laugh, and then they'll get on no matter what. There are people who really work, but maybe they've got a bit of a funny accent. I know that sounds stupid but the police are so childish and petty when you think of these people, fully grown adults it's so daft. I don't know, maybe there is something about an officer which looks a bit strange or maybe the relief thinks he's even queer; I mean it doesn't matter, but maybe they think that and they will give them such a hard time.

Nor is it necessary for the new recruit to have actual experience of coming up against group reaction to know what the reaction would be to a certain eventuality; the initiate quickly learns the boundaries of acceptable and unacceptable behaviour, attitudes and perspectives:

It's like if you're sitting in the canteen and you read a book you'll get some comment; people will take the mickey because you're reading a book. If you're reading some *stupid* book that would be all right. I mean, if I went into the canteen and sat there reading *Playboy*, if I got any comments it would be either people having a look or things that would bolster my self-esteem, like being a popular thing to do – not that it's done, but I know that it would be, right? But if you sit down and read a book on some aspect of law, an intellectual book, you're bound to get some comments. If you come in reading the *Sun*, no-one's gonna say 'ah you're reading the *Sun*' but if you came in and you was reading the *Guardian* or the *Independent*, someone is bound to pass a comment. Which is just like, over a period, it can change people's personalities in terms of what is expected of them.

The socialization process is applied to all newcomers to the group, not just to probationer officers, and it may be enforced through 'informal disciplinary' mechanisms as well as by exhortation and social disapproval. It is certainly intensely expressed in big city forces such as the Met., where the group is often constituted by young, male, unattached officers without local connections, living in section houses, whose relationships are social as well as job related. As one London officer put it, in explaining why he was never able to become accepted into the group, 'The relief go drinking of a morning! They go out after night shift to market pubs in the early hours. To me, well, I can't handle it at six o'clock in the morning.' But the process is not confined to big city forces, as was brought home to us by many officers in all three forces studied. Officers spoke of individuals being 'ostracized', of being made 'black sheep', and of being turned into 'loners'. The following extended extract from a Gwent officer displays the full power of group socialization at work there. The officer pointed out that sometimes individuals were transferred to the area who did not fit in; the interview continued:

Q: What happens if you have on the shift an individual who doesn't fit in?

A: Then they won't stay on the shift very long. You have to work together, you've got to co-operate with each other all the time, otherwise you can get all sorts of problems.

Q: If he doesn't fit in, how would the rest of the shift regard him?

A: As an outcast. His life would be hell.

Q: Really?

A: That's what I have found. A person comes on to a shift, they've got to know where he's worked, why he's come to the shift, what's his background, what's his reputation like. So he comes on to our shift. He has to fit in to the ways the shift is run, organized, how you deal with things, who organizes what, what the work rate is. If he doesn't fit in, then any mistakes he'll make will be instantly jumped upon, bitterly criticized and it'll get to the point where he'll probably think he can't do anything right at all. Then he'll ask to go and he'll go. He has to prove himself. He'll probably get the routine work, what we call routine, to begin with, not particularly exciting, and if he can cope with that he'll get accepted. And if he fits in with our sense of humour – it's the strangest type involved but his attitude will have to coincide with the attitude of the shift. If he doesn't fit, his life will be made hell by most of the shift.

Q: How?

A: He'll find himself working differently to most of us, get given different jobs. Just generally made to feel he doesn't fit in. He'll have the piss taken all the time, for want of a better explanation.

Q: Does this test apply to everyone who joins the shift?
A: Yes. It's more or less a clique. If there is a hard core, say three or four of you worked the same shift for a good number of years, they develop a clique situation and you are either in or you are out. It's strange really, I never thought of saying that about the police but it's true.

Established officers were better able to survive such experiences: they had witnessed or undergone this kind of treatment themselves and had developed coping mechanisms. These ranged from securing autonomy through attachment to one of the specialist squads (which tend to have even greater internal solidarity) or to community beat work, or negotiating a presence that was acceptable to the rest of the group by not overtly contesting the established norms of perspective and behaviour. Some spoke of having to overcome 'bad probationary reports' or the attachment of labels which could have inhibited progress ('I was labelled as quiet and shy because I didn't join in their comments and racist attitudes') and several officers spoke eloquently of the constant and overarching problem of dealing with their colleagues as being a priority consideration, as with the following officer:

Q: Tell me about your experiences on the relief.
A: I do know one thing, I could never ever treat people the way I have seen some people be treated, and go home and sleep like a baby at night. I just couldn't do that. I couldn't go home knowing I've hurt someone, not intentionally and not in the way that I know some people laugh and really enjoy hurting someone.
Q: Is this hurting each other as police officers or people in the community?
A: I'm just talking about the police. It's just some of the relief politics, as it's referred to, it is ridiculous. Yet at the same time I understand it, but I just couldn't do and say and treat some of the people like they do get treated. That's why in a million years I never dreamed it would be like that, and never ever thought there would be much worry for people because of that side. I would say most of the stress is because of that, from other colleagues and not because of what is happening on the streets. . . . The only thing that bothers me is other colleagues, and not the street. It's sometimes an excuse. I think that the stress on police is because of all the

people they deal with; I don't think it is so much. I'd say there is stress sometimes possibly with going to court, it can be quite worrying. Doesn't matter how much service you've got, it's just nervousness because you don't know what's happening. I mean I sort of worry about that but I think most of the stress comes from other colleagues, I really do.

Greater difficulties are experienced by new recruits. Some are driven out of the police, as is reported to be the case with young officers from ethnic minorities (for example *The Observer*, 12 November 1989), while others, as van Maanen (1977) notes, try to shed the 'rookie' label by various means of transcending their station including 'taking on more responsibility than permissible, ingratiating [themselves] with superiors, making pretentious use of local argot or even behaving vituperatively toward other newcomers'. The following interview with a relief officer exemplifies these points:

Q: How did you find trying to get accepted by the relief?
A: Difficult, I would say worrying as well. You've got to get accepted, it's your main worry. It's ridiculous, you come into work worrying about whether other people will accept you on the relief. I look back and think of some of the things I did just to get accepted. You know, it might be something daft like buying someone a coffee or something like that, or running around trying to help them with paperwork. It wasn't because I was particularly keen and wanted to do the paperwork, more that I wanted to be accepted and liked. . . .
Q: How were you made to feel?
A: Nothing was done to me that was criminal or bad or anything like that. There was probably a lot of chat behind my back and all that kind of stuff, but maybe that was just me being sensitive. Again some people don't worry about it; and some of that was unnecessary, looking back on some of the idiots I know who said things like that, who I think are totally useless and really lazy. I can't believe I just accepted it and let it go into my head. . . .
Q: So how do you feel, that you have to. . .?
A: Awful! Honestly I went home sometimes and I was in tears, it doesn't matter saying it does it? But some of the people I've seen. . . . I've seen one particular person destroyed and did leave the police force and my opinion is, hasn't said it to

me, but my opinion is that it was that he didn't get enough
help from his colleagues and he couldn't cope. Couldn't
cope with the mickey taking and things that were happening
to him.

The collective effect on new members who survive induction, is to
equip them with 'a set of rules, perspectives, prescriptions, techniques, and/or tools necessary' for them to continue as participants
in the organization (van Maanen, 1974, p. 81). As Fielding points
out, these career perspectives are not concerned directly with the
practicalities of everyday practice but instead 'with long-range,
occupationally relevant orientations. They provide an "operating"
*ideology* which assists constables in developing a conception of who
they are and what they are to do' (1988b, p. 16, original emphasis).

### Community service versus law enforcement

The maintenance of this broad ideology, described in Chapter 6,
is assisted by the structural divide between relief officers and those
responsible for community beat work. This segmentation of police
work represents much more than a mere division of labour between short-term, fast-response, fire-brigade policing, and
long-term, community policing; rather it symbolizes the continued
commitment to fire-brigade policing as the central mode of delivering policing and the rejection of the appropriateness of
community policing as a viable core activity. Indeed, relief officers
see the existence of CBOs as *legitimating* relief styles, by supplying
the 'public relations bit' and satisfying a public demand for beat
officers.

[CBOs] are put in a difficult position where they are trying to
be nice to a community and they have also got the job of trying
to arrest people. Whereas the relief doesn't necessarily have to
earn that respect because he doesn't meet these people every
day on his beat.

The idea of home beats in an [inner-city] area like this, I have
got severe reservations about; it's not a homogenous area,
people are continually on the move, there isn't a community
spirit here at all, they are all small groups, very small groups of
people, who represent all sorts of factions but the idea of the
village bobby is a non-starter in a vast majority of areas like this.

However, if we don't at least try to place some format of policing as far as that is concerned we would be left with purely an army of occupation and that clearly is something which I wouldn't like to see.

Similarly, CBOs see it as part of their core function to paper over the failings of relief officers and to present the acceptable face of policing.

I find myself constantly having to try and smooth over instances that've occurred where they might have had a burglary and a relief officer's gone down there and, understandably being a relief officer, being very pressured . . . he's in and out as quickly as he can: 'What happened? What's been taken? How did they get in? Ta ta, bye bye.' I get a lot of reports back from people saying 'He didn't seem very interested. He was only there five minutes. Didn't even ask me name . . .'

I don't think the lads on relief realise how many times we brush people down and say 'Well, you know, give the bloke a break, he's probably had a bad day. . . .' As a [CBO] you are there more as a mediator between the public and the police.

The broad policing ideology which favours law enforcement over community service is also held in position by the reward and assessment systems within the police organization. The way in which officers are assessed from the moment of admission to the probationary ranks teaches them the kinds of behaviour which will attract official approval and instils in most officers an under-standing of what needs to be done in order to secure a place in a specialist squad, promotion or, at the most basic level, a 'quiet life' free from the criticisms of supervisors. The initiate learns very quickly that assessment within the police is a simple matter: 'figures'. Whilst probationers understand the need to gain experi-ence in all aspects of policing and that issuing summonses and making arrests are an essential part of this experience, the training period instils in officers the *centrality* of these activities. It also teaches officers that the production of crime figures should take precedence over other policing objectives such as forging good relations with the community, as the following probationer illus-trates:

The other thing, I think, is that generally there is – the management won't say this – when you're a probationer and when you're first out of your probation you are under pressure to produce figures. They'll tell you there is no numbers game, but there is. You have a six-monthly report written and each time it's numbers, numbers, numbers; how many arrests have you made, how many processes have you done, how many this, how many that. Therefore, instead of the PC approaching a particular incident with a mind to saying 'Well, what I'm gonna do is just give him a good talking to and let him go' he automatically gets his book out and he starts writing. You will gain a lot more support perhaps . . . I'm not saying you've got to butter up the public, but it won't always be necessary to get the pen and start writing. But because you're under pressure for numbers and it looks good on your report that you done x number of processes, you can't come in and say 'Well, I didn't stick him on because I felt that it was a better result just to tell him off.'

The emphasis upon arrests and summonses, known through each force as 'the numbers game' or 'process races', is an embedded feature of policing, officers told us, which affected the kind of policing they were prepared to undertake. Outside Gwent, officers who wanted attachment to a specialist squad such as CID, for example, told us that their chances of transfer were absolutely dependent upon the quantity and quality of their arrests. This led many officers to reject CB work altogether and to stay instead on relief work, further contributing to the stigmatization of community beat work as not involving real policing. In turn, CBOs were usually unable to transfer directly to specialist squads but had to return first to the relief in order to 'get the arrests first' because it was understood *and accepted as appropriate* that arrests should be the basis of the decision: 'If you want to go to the crime squad or something then they will look at your arrests, nothing else, which is fair enough.'

Moreover, the pressure for results affected the way in which CBOs discharged their responsibilities. Setting aside the social pressure from their relief counterparts to engage in 'real' work rather than 'just drinking tea', many CBOs in Avon and Somerset and Gwent in particular felt under direct pressure from their superiors to generate crime figures. In this way, officers felt that the 'numbers game' directly undercut community policing objectives, represented a standing pressure on CBOs, and put in jeopardy their relations with the local community. The following interview extracts from Gwent and Avon and Somerset CBOs illustrate these conflicts:

*Avon and Somerset*
The crime figures are looked at, scrutinized, and if we have got a low detection rate they think 'what are they all doing in [his area]?' When somebody from Headquarters looks at what is going on, he doesn't know all the good work I am doing that is not related to crime.

A CBO is not assessed by what he should be doing – 'forging links with the community'. In fact, the people who would be assessing him aren't prone to assessing in that respect at all. They're prone to assessing in other ways, by the amount of paperwork he's putting in, what sort of quality his paperwork is, what his appearance is. There's a section on the staff appraisal form about how he's thought of by other members of his group, but there's nothing on there to say how he's thought of by the people he serves.

The fault of the system is when senior officers measure success with crime detection rates. The way they have been brought up you can measure success on crime prevention rates, which is totally wrong, but it's the way the system works.

*Gwent*
To be quite honest I don't think senior officers know what's going on. Because they don't know what you're doing. You don't come in and say 'I've been up to see Mrs Jones today', or whatever. You just carry on with the job quietly. They tend to look at how effective you are from results. People you've booked, crimes you've detected, figures, statistics. If at the end of the day you weren't providing any statistics at all you wouldn't find yourself being a [CBO] long or, realistically, in the police force very long. They'd certainly want to make you conform to a standard that they think is obtainable, which means upholding the law in their eyes.

They judge whether you are doing a good job on figures. The only way anything is assessed in this job is on figures, process figures, crime figures.

I find that if I have got an hour or a couple of hours to myself, where maybe I'd like to go and chat to someone in the street and then maybe go into the house, I'm unable to do it because you've got pressure, not pounding down your neck all the time, but you're thinking 'I haven't booked anybody today', or 'I haven't booked anybody for two or three days, I'd better go out and look for someone', when you know you're going out and basically you're hounding the motorist because you want to stop them, you're looking for offences on the vehicle to come back and you put it in the book to say 'well, yes, I haven't just been walking the street all day, I have been stopping cars', when really in areas like this perhaps you should be talking to people a bit more, especially youngsters.

## SITUATED WORK PRACTICES

Police occupational culture is not, however, simply a product of the internal dynamics of the group or even of the legacy of the collective experiences of officers in the past. Rather, police sub-culture is forged and re-forged in situated work practices, in the daily encounters with citizens as officers go about their work. Just as each positive interaction with one of the 'respectables' reaffirms the correctness of the identification of the middle class as law-abiding and as supporters of the police, every negative encounter with the 'roughs' vindicates accepted police typologies. Indeed, the police have such faith in their own classification system that 'reverse encounters' of either kind are written off as aberrational or used to confirm the essential 'fairness' of their policing practices. In this way, situated work practices reproduce in intense ways police typologies. Whilst our data show this to be a feature of police dealings with white working-class communities today as it has been in the past (Storch, 1975; Cohen, P., 1979; Davis, 1989), in our study this can be best seen in relation to the inner-city areas in London and Bristol, where police encounters with members of the ethnic minority communities only serve to deepen and entrench police racism.

The police do not evidence a simple pathological dislike and suspicion of young black people, but mistrust and dislike them in specific ways. Contrary to popular imagination, policing is not often concerned with the enforcement of law, and if it were, we could expect the police to be much more active in prosecution-terms than they currently are. In all the areas in which they patrol, officers see infractions of the law which could be punished but which, for a variety of reasons, they choose not to punish. This is true of 'black' areas as well of 'white' areas. However, officers hold, as we have seen, a much more negative view of black people which cannot simply be attributed to any greater lawlessness. Instead, it is related to another, and central, aspect of policing, namely, the *affirmation of authority*. When officers walk through white suburban roads, whether people tell them that it is 'nice to see a constable' or complain about the infrequency of patrols police authority is thereby acknowledged. In black areas especially, however, the deference and respect which the police demand is not forthcoming, and is replaced by actions which contest their authority and subject individual officers to ridicule and abuse:

> The main problem for the PC in the street is the lack of respect from the majority of the [black] community, the lack of co-operation.

> They are hostile towards us. The looks, I know it's all personal interpretation but we can all tell a dirty look from a pleasing one and the sounds they make you know like the, it's mostly the young, the young generally coloured you'd have to say and just the young, I'll try not to use police terms now, but the young just very . . . the sort of 'slaggy' types that, be they white or black they are going to look upon you in some derisory manner and they'll make their customary silly noises and things, like teeth-sucking and say things and call you stupid names like, well just mutter it under their breath, like 'blood clot' and all that rubbish they speak. There's plenty of that I would say yeah. Just a general sort of total lack of respect. . .

The police demand for deference is well attested in the literature on policing (Chevigny, 1969; Reiss, 1971; Lee, 1981) and absence of deference is interpreted by the police as a challenge to their authority (Fink and Sealy, 1974). In the case of black people, however, the lack of deference is seen to come from a culture which itself is anti-authority, which in turn comes from countries which are disorganized and ill disciplined. And so the racist chain goes on.

## The black 'challenge' to police authority

Apart from failing to show deference, black people are also seen directly to challenge police authority. They are seen to do this because they contest the legitimacy of police actions or their fairness, accusing officers of discriminatory selection or discriminatory treatment.

> If you stop someone round here, they'll argue about the silliest little things. Always answer you back and stuff. I'm not saying they'll hit you or anything, but there is a lot of abuse and people say you're picking on them because you're white and they're black and so on. I'm not just picking on one group, blacks or white or whatever. All people you stop, especially young people who've been involved with crime before, don't treat you with any respect and will swear at you and say you are picking on them because of their colour. With the black and white thing, it's a no-win situation.

> You can stop them because they are in a car and there is something about the car that you don't like or the person that's driving it and you just want to speak to them. I mean I'm generally pleasant at the beginning anyway. Immediately they are on to you, they start shouting and swearing and coming at you. It's very difficult not to say anything back; and you do sometimes because you just, you know, it gets ridiculous.

Where police action is thought necessary or desirable, therefore, it is on the basis that the citizen will take objection to it and the officer will be unable to convince the individual of the fairness of the action. Black people, in this representation, cannot be convinced of the fairness of police behaviour because they will not listen to reason:

> The criminal element down [here] – there's no way you can reason with them. They make it blatantly obvious that they hate you for a start, you're not wanted in the area. There's absolutely no way in a million years of seeing any sense in talking to them. I mean, you can't say 'put your seatbelt on', you can't do that because they consider that they don't have to do that, that you shouldn't be talking to them in that way.

> Certainly some of them are extremely difficult to deal with, they seem to go out of their way to go against any form of authority.

The only thing they seem to understand is to be arrested. Why this is I don't know, but it is a fact that a percentage are extremely difficult to deal with. They don't listen to what you say even when you are helping them; they're still complaining.

The consequence is that there is a police propensity to arrest rather than to stand and argue the matter on the street. But since black people are seen by the police as aggressive and prone to violence, and since black communities are seen to be mutually protective and willing to combine to frustrate police action, the police favour 'snatch' arrests, grabbing suspected offenders and removing them from the area as quickly as possible, before any crowd can gather or any other violence occur. Officers from both Avon and Somerset and the Met. explained that this could be seen by onlookers as 'aggressive policing', whilst acknowledging that the style adopted could and did produce a ratchet effect on violence:

People get so aggressive with searches they end up becoming arrested for public order matters and immediately you get more problems, you know: 'I was stopped in the street, I didn't like it and they arrested me for nothing'. It's immediate, all this goes on and on and on and it's so frustrating. Although I never thought I could, I don't agree with it at all, but I never thought I could understand why people get punched, why people end up with massive complaints about punching somebody in the face about this, that and the other; I can see why it happens. It's a steady, steady build up, it just happened to be one incident out there after ten years of stress, and they just make you click, especially working in a sensitive area. You go to work some days and you just haven't got the patience that day to deal with them; and they can be, it can be a very, very difficult job. Really you are in conflict with them the majority of the time.

Because of the absence of positive police–citizen relations and the perceived potential for violence towards the police in these areas, policing is usually conducted by pairs or groups of officers. Whilst this may be an understandable protective strategy, it too has a tendency to increase the likelihood of aggression and violence, a point remarked upon by probationary officers:

The officer you are with might say things, make comments or be rude. As a probationer, the only way you are going to get involved noticeably in that situation is to go in *heavier* than the

officer who's just gone in: he's spoken to him and there's no way
I'm going to be able to; he's already having a go at him, so you
can't get involved by being polite because your voice is going to
be drowned out. Rather than get involved by being low key, the
only way you are going to get involved noticeably is by getting
right stuck in and being more aggressive than you know, [push
aside] that officer, say 'I'm going to talk to him' and be *more*
aggressive. (original emphasis)

The tendency toward aggression and over-reaction is given impetus by the failure of the police to establish links with the
community which would allow anything resembling 'normal' relations to prevail. From the community viewpoint, there can be no
trust in the police even in periods of police inactivity because these,
it is known, will be broken by raids or other aggressive incursions.
From the police viewpoint, periods of inactivity are 'enforced' by
senior officers who want to keep the lid on and avoid 'uprisings'
before they move on to another posting. These policies build up
resentment in the rank and file who are denied the routine work
upon which they rely and who consequently see the black districts
as virtual 'no-go' areas:

> You can't stop a vehicle because they won't stop. So all the
> traffic-type process goes out the window. That was your bread
> and butter type offences – one headlight, through a red traffic
> light, things like that that you do just to keep you ticking over,
> you just don't do at all if you're in that area. Once you take away
> traffic there's very little other offences you can actually get to
> grips with. You got the occasional bill poster you can report for
> summons. You wouldn't report anyone for walking a dog
> without a lead because no-one has leads on dogs down there,
> and you wouldn't report anyone for litter.

> Especially as a probationer, you stop ropey vehicles because you
> look for traffic offences, the bread and butter of a policeman
> basically. Now, you stop such vehicles in most places, although
> some people can be upset when they're stuck on for an offence,
> at the end of the day you're not going to see any serious
> problems with that. But certainly in the main part of [this area]
> if you start stopping ropey vehicles with young Afro-Caribbean
> males in it you're in for a lot of abuse, verbal abuse, and quite
> possibly, depending on where you stop them and who's about,

a crowd forming and problems that might come from it. And the last thing you want to do really or the last thing that supervisory senior officers at this station want is for people to go over there and continually stop vehicles and cause problems where police officers get injured, vehicles get damaged, and possibly a riot or a mini riot or a serious disorder occurs because of that.

The result is that when action is licensed in these areas it strongly tends towards the sudden, violent and aggressive, and explains why the public, as described in Chapter 2, see inner-city policing in these terms. These are not misconceptions, but reflect only too well a policing character which reaffirms for the police in every enacted encounter the correctness of the world-view celebrated in police subculture.

## THE BONDS OF LOYALTY

At one level, it may seem puzzling to an outsider how the policing ideology and occupational culture of constables can survive in the face of the ever-present risk that an officer out of sympathy with prevailing attitudes and practices will break ranks. It is clear, for example, that some of those to whom we spoke in the course of our research wished to distance themselves from their colleagues, were upset by racist language and behaviour, and were highly critical of unfair or unjust conduct that they had witnessed. Some, indeed, had made their discontent clear by overt challenge in canteen exchanges, or by their general disposition and demeanour. Disaffection was, therefore, apparent in some cases to the rank and file and might be expected, of itself, to act as a restraint on unacceptable behaviour. This, however, would be to seriously misjudge the sacred nature of policing to those involved (Manning, 1977) and to underestimate the bonds of silence which it creates.

The most important thing that probationary officers learn in their first few months in the police is the need to keep their mouths shut about practices, including those in breach of the rules, which experienced officers deem necessary in discharging policing responsibilities. Secrecy and loyalty are enjoined not because the initiates themselves become implicated by their first failure to complain (although on occasions this too can be a central in-

fluence), but because the socialization process teaches probationers to subordinate their own views to the needs and demands of
the job. In other words, the novice 'who survives on the force learns
to look at the world through the needs of his/her occupation' (Lee,
1981, p. 51, citing Vincent, 1979, p. 92 ff., and Bayley and
Mendelsohn, 1968, p. 106). Police culture and ideology is thus
underpinned by a code of secrecy which creates a 'wall of silence'
(Jennings and Lashmar, 1990) which in turn produces cover-up
practices:

> What you are told is that if you get into trouble your governors
> will stick behind you. There is no clarification that what you
> should be doing is *moral*; it's 'Don't worry, we'll stick behind you
> *regardless*.' It's like watching *The Bill*: if you watch that they are
> trying to project some of the attitudes and values you get in the
> police but watching it, it doesn't actually match what the police
> is like at all. Like when a PC does something – like last night on
> TV a particular member of the CID was involved in something
> where a juvenile jumped off a roof, got injured and the rest of
> the programme was all about the grief he was receiving from
> senior officers, even his sergeant saying 'Oh no, maybe it was
> your fault'. Whereas there would never ever be that pressure at
> all: there's too much 'you all stick together' rather than a whole
> air of suspicion being created. Even if it was suspicious there
> would be an air of 'Oh, how can we cover this up?' I'm not saying
> they'd say 'Oh, how can we cover this up?'; it's subtle.

Secrecy is then 'a protective armour shielding the force as a whole
from public knowledge of infractions' (Reiner, 1985, p. 93) and all
the officers to whom we spoke accepted the sacredness of the
loyalty principle. This principle applies not only to minor indis-
cretions but also to infractions of a potentially serious kind as well
as to plainly criminal behaviour, as the following two examples
illustrate.

The first, drawn from Avon and Somerset, was provided by an
experienced officer who stressed to us the centrality of 'peer
loyalty' as an organizing principle of group policing ('You stick up
for that PC to outside bodies but within the station you'd say "He's
bloody useless, isn't he?"'). Illustrating this loyalty principle, he
recounted an occasion on which a fellow constable had committed
a serious assault on a citizen, gratuitously punching him in the

sight of other officers. He stressed that the account had to 'remain suitably vague' in order to protect identities:

> There's a policeman having belted this bloke, several times, and, ah, it was witnessed by several officers one of whom was very young in service, very nervous and knew what he had seen. All the others had a bit more service and knew all the things that could result; this police officer in my opinion would have been sent down, even though the injuries weren't that substantial. . . . If you know the officer well, if he's been a policeman friend of yours, are you really going to send him down? The officer who had been fighting, if it was the other way round, would they turn round about their mate and say 'Yes, he hit the police officer', so you find yourself perhaps thinking in terms of their rules, which are the ones you are up there to stand against.
>
> The younger officer was, to a large extent with his best interests at heart, persuaded that he couldn't really have seen what he thought he saw, which provided him with an opportunity to withdraw with honour, from initially saying 'I saw it and I'm standing firm' to 'Oh, you are quite right; if I'm standing there, I couldn't really have seen it, could I?' And I don't know, it was out of order; I told the bloke who it was, it was out of order but giving evidence against him, seeing him go to prison for fighting in a way you do with fights dozens and dozens of times a year, I don't know.

> (After the tape-recorder was switched off, the officer tearfully confessed that he was the officer who had persuaded the 'young officer' to withdraw his original account. He said that he had reconciled his position in his mind by telling the sergeant that he would never again work with the officer who had carried out the assault.)

We see in this account the power of peer loyalty displayed in two ways. On the positive side is the respondent's affirmation that protection of a colleague comes above the duty to uphold the law, a duty that is plain to the officer in his recognition that his actions are consistent only with 'street', not legal or moral, rules. On the negative side is the absolute nature of the loyalty principle, breach of which will lead to ostracism by colleagues and a blight on or end to a police career, as seen by his well-founded assertion that he was motivated towards the young officer 'with his best interests at heart'.

The second example is derived from a Metropolitan officer's account of his time as a driver of a support unit van. Vans of this kind, which may contain a sergeant and up to a dozen or so constables, are essentially mobile reserve units offering extra cover at scenes of major incidents. Historically, these vans, often deployed in areas with large ethnic minority populations and utilizing para-military policing tactics, have attracted bitter criticism, with the notorious Special Patrol Group (SPG) seen as 'an elite, aggressive, unaccountable squad, known for its involvement in public order confrontations' (Kettle and Hodges, 1982, p. 93. See also Rollo, 1980; Scarman, 1981; Benyon, 1984; Ward, 1986). Indiscriminate road blocks and other stop and search tactics, bullying, intimidation of bystanders and confrontational methods have been said to characterize interventions by such mobile reserve units, as well as the unprovoked assaults which marked the notorious 'Holloway Road incident' in which boys walking along the roadside were beaten up by members of a passing patrol van (East, 1987; Hilliard, 1987). The existence of such vans, and the policing practices associated with their members, attracted – it will be recalled from Chapter 2 above – strident and spontaneous public criticism from residents in both the Met. and Avon and Somerset. In our field-work interviews a Metropolitan officer described how the cadre of officers in his van persistently engaged in 'inappropriate' and 'incorrect' behaviour. These officers spent a great deal of time waiting for something to happen and, to relieve the boredom, acted in a disparaging, provocative and threatening manner towards members of the public. He continued:

> I was the driver and I didn't like the attitude of the vast majority of people on the van. I didn't think the sergeant had any control over them. They were pulling silly pranks and not behaving in a professional manner.
>
> One evening, I wasn't in a very good frame of mind and their pranks just got too silly. There was nothing cruel or dangerous. They were just being idiots. Cat-calling out the window at females, and they were ribbing me because I wasn't joining in. On my way to a call which we weren't going to get to – I mean, the sergeant said 'go' but I knew full well that we'd be called off before we got there; it was too far – it just got to me. I stopped

in the middle of the road, blue light going round, put the handbrake on, picked up my cap and put it on my head, opened the door and walked off.

Now, of course, that sergeant could have disciplined me, he could have reported me. The following morning I walked in to the canteen and I said 'You and I had better talk. You can do me for discipline if you want but you're coming with me, because you're getting up to all sorts of stupidity and you know it. I shall spill the lot. Or we can just go to the governor and say "Look, it doesn't suit me. I'd like to go back to my old duties"', which is what happened.

In this account we see how discreditable behaviour by a tight-knit group of officers can continue notwithstanding the presence of a 'supervising officer', and how that behaviour and the extraordinary response of the driver are both insulated from external scrutiny by the overarching code of loyalty. Together with other accounts of the demands of loyalty, it underlines the courage of officers who are willing to implicate their colleagues in misdeeds. Such officers – whose careers may be thereby ruined – display extraordinary resolution. For officers of normal firmness of mind, however, loyalty in this setting is blind.

## THE INFLUENCE OF 'CONTROL' SYSTEMS

Even if rank and file police culture is characterized by a strong independent and autonomous propensity, shielded by networks of understanding and codes of secrecy, it still remains to be asked why it appears immune to any 'civilizing' tendencies of management, because there can be no doubt that senior management has occasionally displayed a commitment (and not only at a rhetorical level) to a more positive style of policing. Thus, for example, following persistent criticisms of racism within the police, the Metropolitan Police Commissioner, Sir David McNee, commissioned an independent study of policing in 1979 which was conducted by the Policy Studies Institute. Before the study was completed, Sir David expressed the hope that the results would 'assist the Metropolitan Police in formulating its strategy for the rest of the decade and beyond' (*Sunday Mirror*, 7 November 1982). The results of this study, revealing deep racism, sexism and stereotyping within the police, were greeted with dismay but also with a renewed commitment to change.

Since then, however, attempts to strengthen 'community involvement', to attract members of ethnic minorities into the police, and to combat racism within the force have not met with significant success. Indeed, in 1989 the Commissioner, Sir Peter Imbert, ordered a top-level inquiry into the treatment of black officers in his force in the face of increased resignations among ethnic minorities and falling recruitment (*The Observer*, 12 November 1989). This followed an earlier study undertaken by Wolff Ohlins in 1988 which found that officers were alienating the public by aggressive, rude and unhelpful behaviour, and which in turn generated a new 'Plus Programme', the heart of which was an attempt to give primacy to 'customer service' (*Guardian*, 21 February 1990). There is evidence of a serious dialogue with many of the values of traditional policing cultures: the recent decision to treat civil disputes with a racial element as possible criminal offences in order to send 'subliminal messages' to officers (*Guardian*, 20 October 1990); the Police Complaints Authority's intent to start recording allegations of racially discriminatory behaviour by officers (*Guardian*, 16 October 1990); new recruitment drives by various forces to attract ethnic minority recruits (*Guardian*, 13 March 1990 and 31 August 1990); new 'mentor' schemes to retain ethnic minority recruits (*Guardian*, 1 November 1990); the acceptance by the Metropolitan Police that ethnic minority recruits were discouraged from staying in the police by the racism of white officers (*The Observer*, 18 November 1990); and the publication of a new statement of common purpose by the Association of Chief Police Officers emphasizing a shift from law enforcement towards 'reassurance policing' (*Guardian*, 14 October 1990). To date, however, that culture has remained broadly intact and we need to explain its continued vitality.

A fundamental point to make is that the broad context which permits the emergence of a forceful policing subculture is the *legal* one (Brogden *et al.*, 1988, p. 34). This is characterized by 'the doctrine of constabulary independence on the one hand . . . and discretion in law enforcement on the other' (pp. 34–5). Legal rules and doctrine are so organized that they accord operational officers maximum discretion (whether to take official action, whether to arrest, whether to charge), and attempts to control the rank and file continually have to contend with the 'political space' accorded individual officers. Legal doctrine is also ambiguous and often increases the uncertainty of officers about how their actions will be officially viewed, an uncertainty which throws them back on to the group and its protective canopy. In addition to this, officers learn from the outset of their career that 'you can't do it by the book', that 'you can only learn from experienced officers out on the street'. A key feature of occupational culture, therefore, dictates suspicion of book rules, and promotes reliance upon the peer group with its associated codes of loyalty and secrecy. Once officers move away from the group, the basis of trust is lost. This is especially true in respect of management and its associated disciplinary and reward structures, as officers from all forces made clear to us:

*Avon and Somerset officer*
If I went to a superintendent and told him what I've told you on anything, I would probably live in fear and trepidation. . . . He's there to enforce some form of discipline on you. That's the way the job is – to try and catch you out.

*Gwent officer*
No matter what they say, if they say 'We'll talk off the record' it can never be off the record with them. It will always be thrown back at you. Because of that you are always on your guard.

*Metropolitan officer*
If you have a problem, I'd be wary of things which would affect my job because whatever [management] say to you, it is all written down.

In addition to the legal context there is, therefore, a specifically organizational context, exemplified by Cain in the following passage:

If a 'war on crime' is demanded, and bureaucratic evidence of success in the form of arrest or clear up rates, then infringement of the rules in order to achieve these objectives becomes an occupational necessity. Not only is illegality (police primary deviance) engendered, but also secondary deviance in terms of secretiveness, and the formation of close-knit, self-protective colleague organization which makes secrecy possible. Such an organization renders the police as impervious to exhortation from the top of their own hierarchy as to the requirements of courts, lawyers, and concerned members of the public.

(Cain, 1979, p. 146)

A legal context which provides freedom to work, and a work context which emphasizes the importance of 'subversive' situated behaviour combine against managerial influence. That influence is further reduced by rank and file distinctions between 'governors' and 'bosses', and by their general conceptions of 'management'.

## Governors, bosses and butterfly men

Within the ranks there is a general divide between immediate supervisory staff – 'governors', and officers of higher ranks – 'bosses'. Governors, who are essentially constituted by the shift sergeant and inspector (but may include senior managers seen as 'good'), are in daily touch with the ranks, work their shifts and share their travails. They are judged on the basis of their personal qualities and their practical skills. To get along with the shift and to influence their work patterns, governors need to have a personable manner, be willing to participate in street-level activity, understand the demands and stresses of the job, and make things as tolerable as possible for the ranks by adjusting work patterns and permitting 'easing' practices. Good governors are sensitive to the subtleties of policing and can get the best out of their officers by small adjustments, as this Gwent officer shows:

> If you have a bad sergeant, in my opinion, the bad sergeant is briefing you, out you get, walk the beat, and all he has you doing is walking that beat for eight hours which at 3.00 a.m., pouring with rain, is a pain in the arse. Whereas in my opinion, if it's a good sergeant he would say, 'OK have a walk about in your sleep for the first couple of hours when there's a lot of people about and then I'll get a car driver to pick you up and have a drive round for a bit, stop a few vehicles or whatever, do what you want'. So basically your night is broken up. 'Later on, say 3.00 a.m., if you team up with so and so, I want you to check the lockups in such and such an area.' If there's two of you, you can pass the time far more quickly than if there's one of you. At 3.00 a.m. there's nowhere to go, there's no one to talk to on your own. I consider you do the job better. If there's one of you,

you might say 'I'm blowed if I am going to walk down there, check that's in order', whereas if there's two of you, you walk down there.

Good governors, then, identify with the ranks, work with them, and fight their corner. Good governors get *implicated* in the activities of the ranks. A good governor may pick up an officer on some mistake but will not make this a public issue, taking that officer aside and speaking about the matter privately. Good governors do not uncritically associate themselves with new force policies but negotiate their impact with their men. Good governors are a part of, not apart from, their officers and will inspire loyalty and respect:

> There was a governor [at an adjacent station] who got posted recently. I mean, I've never heard so many people sing his praise. His turn out for his party was fabulous. And everybody meant it; they were sorry to see him go because he was a *copper*; he was out on the streets with his lads. If anything went wrong he was there with them. He made a decision, whether it was right or wrong, and he thought it was the right one. Afterwards if it was the wrong one he was big enough to turn round and say 'Yeah, I made a mistake!'. And he would *protect his relief*. He'd stick up for his relief. He wouldn't let them get trod on. Now that's the sort of governor you want. (original emphasis)

Properly analysed, therefore, governors are not concerned with general police policy but instead are to be understood in terms of morale. They are one of the critical influences upon the spirit of the relief, setting an atmosphere which motivates officers or, in the case of bad governors, generating disgruntlement and resentment.

By contrast, the police subculture presents 'bosses' as divorced from real policing. 'Management cops', as Reiner (1985, p. 43) points out, are derided by 'street-wise' operational officers. In the eyes of the rank and file, the gulf between the two results from the transformational effects on the person of becoming a manager and from the different functions of the two levels. So far as constables are concerned, the promotion process transforms people from 'officers' into 'managers' or 'bosses'. In this conception, a manager is distinguished by having no understanding of the demands of street-level policing, of the changes which have taken place since the time when they were officers. We found, as had Kinsey (1985), that constables saw such senior officers as remote from police work. In our samples of officers, whilst almost one-half of those in Gwent made positive evaluations of senior management, this was true in the other two forces only of one-quarter of officers. According to the rank and file, managers are 'out of touch':

*Avon and Somerset officer*
The management have no idea of what the police force on the ground is like nowadays. None whatsoever. They have not done it for years and years and years. They have no idea of the type of work that we have to do, the frustrations, the type of public we are dealing with, the general resentment that is felt towards the police, here and there, they just do not know what it is like. Whereas I could picture myself sat behind a desk and I could experience what a senior officer's job is all about, reading through files and such like and making decisions, I am the person on the street who has to make an instant decision whether to arrest somebody. Whatever I do I have even more of a decision making role than he has to play.

*Gwent officer*
Once you get to the rank of inspector you are not a policeman, you are a civilian in uniform. You can have senior officers with only twelve months' experience on the street. They can retain knowledge out of a book, but out on the street they haven't got a bloody clue.

*Metropolitan officer*
My immediate sort of governors, inspectors and so forth are very very helpful to me. They can do no wrong really. But above that level they are out of touch. I mean the last time they were operational in the front line it might have been somewhere like Surbiton anyway. They've sort of, once you get to the rank of sergeant it's pretty easy to duck and dive especially if you are at a nice nick. And once you're an inspector well that's it, you can sit in all day and just sit in an office. Really these people might not have walked the beat or dealt with situations we have to deal with on a daily basis; it's probably totally alien to them because they never had to deal with anything like this. In any case people were much nicer, what, fifteen to twenty years ago when they were operational policemen you know.

Greatest scorn is reserved for those 'who have never been in touch'. These are the graduate entrants, known in police argot as 'fliers' or 'butterfly officers'. The introduction of graduate entry schemes and accelerated promotion schemes have produced deep conflicts within the police. Graduates, who constituted only 0.1 per cent (168 officers) of the police in 1968 but some 5.4 per cent (6,625 officers) by 1988, have attracted the resentment of other police officers (Smithers *et al.*, 1990) and have become a focus of concern within organized policing circles. The Police Federation, for example, has attacked 'butterfly' officers who move from job to job in different parts of the country without gaining sufficient experience or building community links (*Police*, 24 August 1989).

In our research, criticisms of this character were common in all forces. Graduate entrants were distinguished by their 'book-learning' and their lack of knowledge of street-level policing: 'Often they don't know what they are doing. They know what the book says they should be doing; but what the book says and how the job is done are quite different – same as any job.' Although there was widespread concern, there was particular resentment shown by the ranks in the inner-city stations of Avon and Somerset and the Met. These stations experienced very rapid turnover of senior officers as they were 'blooded' on inner-city policing before moving on and up the promotion ladder. The following comments give a flavour of the views of rank and file officers on these issues:

A lot of the bosses nowadays are playboys, they are degree men; they are not policemen. They are career men who are in the police force to get as high as they can as quickly as they can. When I joined, a lot of the senior officers were policeman who had started on the ground, who had done their time as PCs, they had done their time as sergeants, done their time as inspectors, they were basically policemen with pips on their shoulder. Nowadays they tend to be academics with pips on their shoulders, and not policemen. We are going more and more that way. . . . It's bad for morale, it's got to be bad for policing in general at the end of the day. If you have got animosity within a force you are not pulling in the same direction, so it has an adverse effect.

The bosses, they are the butterfly men. They're not interested in us as PCs, they are interested in their next move. They are not going to make any decision that's going to jeopardise their next move.

When I joined the force, most supervising officers had a lot of experience, grass-roots experience, probably done ten years as a PC, and then been promoted to sergeant for five–six years, then on to inspector; and finished service after thirty years and haven't been far removed from the job for any length of time. But now with the advent of graduate entries you're finding that there are promotions very early in service and consequently no grass-roots experience and senior officers very often become managers rather than police officers who are supervising. It will suffer over time. Some of these people have never been in touch; many wouldn't know what was happening on the street. If you get an instruction from an officer who you respect, it's far easier to carry out that instruction than it is from someone who you haven't got that respect for as a policeman but you respect their rank obviously.

'Management cops' are not only differentiated from 'street cops' by background and training, but also by function. In the eyes of rank and file, management are there to deal with the public, to project an image of policing in conformity with liberal democratic ideals of egalitarian justice (Shearing, 1981b, p. 31). This involves management in 'PR', in 'selling a line', in 'keeping the lid on'. It also involves, as Shearing (1981b) points out, the systematic denial of the 'reality' of police work as understood by the rank and file. Our officers confirmed this:

When you listen to senior management, not so much talking to us but what we hear them saying through the press because we don't tend to talk to them personally, it's what the middle class majority wants to hear. When the Commissioner makes a statement, it's something that is really again just to satisfy the educated majority who read the newspapers, but all of their ideas are really manufactured for those people.

Management are not actually concerned with policing, what happens in reality. They are concerned with the policies of the area.

Senior officers should back us more. Things – it's like on a press release – are honeyed over: 'I'll cover this one', 'We'll say this and that.' I think senior officers don't stand up for the PCs enough.

This conception of management contributes to the secrecy of the lower ranks which itself enables management to engage in pre-sentational strategies. Whilst rank and file secrecy hides the *details* of deviance from management, it is an overstatement to claim that presentational strategies are conducted 'in real ignorance of what these might cover up' (Reiner, 1985, p. 93). Senior officers have, after all, come up through the ranks and know perfectly well (as many made clear to us) what goes on in terms of the values, ideologies and practices of the rank and file. As they rise through the ranks, however, managerialism distances senior officers from the ranks and encourages them to translate institutional ideologies focused on race and gender into individual bad apples.

So far as the ranks are concerned, management's 'PR' face involves the legitimation of policing not through the denial of reality but through acknowledging it in the disciplining of officers. In their eyes, therefore, this demonstrates the essential hypocrisy of management and its willingness to 'buy favour' at the expense of ordinary constables at times of intense public criticism. It further evidences the gulf between those on the street and those in 'ivory towers' and 'dream factories', and symbolizes the bottom line feeling of the ranks that, when the crunch comes, bosses will not 'stick up' for them.

For reasons which relate to the biographies of bosses as well as their separate functions, therefore, the divide between the ranks and bosses reinforces rather than undercuts police subculture. So far as the ranks are concerned, initiatives which talk of a new 'contract' with the public or a new 'age' of policing are quite independent of the needs and demands of 'real' policing and are more 'sops to the public', dreamed up by senior officers who are increasingly remote from day-to-day policing:

Q: What is your view of the management?
A: We have got a two-tier police force. We have management which is concerned with management concepts and quite clearly over the past few years have made tremendous innovations and changes. We also have a police service which goes out there and deals with the job exactly the same way as it did, or almost the same way as it did, twenty-five years ago. Obviously various rules and regulations have

changed but we are still doing the same thing, going out there, dealing with the problems, day-to-day problems and the two really don't meet. We have a superb management system but it hasn't actually altered what is going on out there.

Q: Is this a source of resentment at ground level?

A: No, because senior management have no, or very little, control or effect on what's happening, certainly from a relief PC's point of view. His line of management structure is his sergeant and his inspector, and rarely will you see anybody above that situation. But as I said it hasn't altered what's done at ground level and really that should be the purpose of any management. If it is trying to change it's not getting to change it, so that it appears to be a cosmetic exercise for outside. It really ought to have an effect on the lower level, that's just where it's failed.

## CONCLUSION

The key features which account for the temper of inner-city policing and the more general aversion towards community policing principles result from institutional attributes of police subculture rather than from the pathologies of individual officers. This police subculture is held in place by networks of understanding and experience transmitted within specific work-group settings which provide officers with a policing ideology. Initiates are, through a mixture of supportive and informal disciplinary mechanisms, rapidly socialized into an occupational culture which teaches them who they are and where they stand. This occupational culture is not detached from social reality but is lived out and 'validated' by situated work practices. It is supported by official reward systems and divisions of labour, held in place by a sacred and overarching code of secrecy, and is reinforced by the ideologies and practices of management. This architecture of police subculture mirrors the wider society, with the less powerful sections the objects of police action and the more powerful the objects of management attempts at legitimation.

# Chapter 8

# Policing communities

Neighbourhood watch appears to be a seductively simple idea. The notion that the police should come together with citizens and form a co-operative agency to promote personal and household security, to deter potential offenders through signs, stickers, and extra vigilance, and to increase the chances of detecting actual or potential offenders through local surveillance activities, seems to provide a mechanism that can be evaluated in its own terms and without considering any wider context. Indeed, much of the 'evaluative' work carried out to date (with the notable exception of Bennett, 1990) has been of this narrow kind (Veater, 1984; O'Leary and Wood, 1984; Anderton, 1985; Northamptonshire Police, 1985). Moreover, much of it has been undertaken by police officers whose positive evaluations of schemes (for example, 'Home Watch is one of the most effective, efficient and successful crime prevention initiatives ever undertaken', Anderton, 1985, p. 53) owe as much to their commitment to the new initative as they do to technical rigour. In this way, the observations of Weatheritt on the general problem of evaluating police innovations are applicable to those which have focused on neighbourhood watch:

> A great deal of discussion of policing innovations has an evangelistic quality to it which makes the innovations unusually difficult to evaluate rationally. This is not difficult to explain. Policing draws its legitimacy from the sacred aspects of tradition and a great deal of . . . policing innovation . . . can be viewed as a reworking of those aspects in new institutional forms. The value of concepts like 'prevention', 'collaborative effort', 'community' and 'public acceptability' lies precisely in their appeal to these sacred aspects: they have a powerful legitimating function. To question the appropriateness of such concepts is thus

to question the legitimacy to which many innovations make appeal and so may appear fundamentally subversive of the very purpose to which they are directed. It is, therefore, hardly surprising that much of the research on policing innovation to date has failed to keep a critical distance from what it sets out to evaluate but has instead become an integral part of the process of legitimating policing activity. In other words, instead of guiding policy, research has conformed to its demands.

(1986, pp. 122–3)

In reviewing neighbourhood watch in the wider context both of public attitudes to crime and the police, and of police attitudes to crime and the public, it is our intention to keep a critical distance from the object of our research. Our concern, it must be emphasized, is not with the alleged failings of individual officers or the shortcomings of individual forces. Nor are we concerned here to create policing typologies, a task which has been undertaken with skill by many other writers (see for example Broderick, 1973; Muir, 1977; Reiner, 1978; Brown, 1981). Rather, we attempt to identify those *structural* features of police organization, police culture, the legal system, and the community, which critically affect the kind of policing delivered and the state of police–community relations.

## THE PUBLIC DEMAND FOR SENSITIVE POLICING

The first point to make is the very close fit, in terms of policing styles and methods, between the promise of neighbourhood watch and the demands of the public. Although it is ironic that the legitimacy of NW rests upon the very same philosophical foundations as the system of policing by car and personal radio it was said to replace, the idea of NW and its associated rhetoric amounts to a rejection of 'technological policing' in which officers are distanced from the public by metal barriers. Putting officers in cars was legitimated on the basis that they would thereby be able to respond more quickly to calls from the public, would be able to spend more time at calls, and could use time that would otherwise be wasted in travelling to deepen relationships within the community. In the new conception, this system is said to have made officers unapproachable and caused them to lose interpersonal skills needed to establish links with the public.

The promise of NW – to provide a system of policing which is both responsive to public demands and sensitive to public needs – is very much in line with the actual wishes of residents. The overwhelming desire of residents is for officers who are friendly and accessible, known to the community, and living in the immediate locality. Whilst residents expect the police to have a fast response capability in answering emergency calls, their other demands are essentially symbolic. The sight of an officer walking the locality provides reassurance, confirming the essential stability of a social order which is rendered problematic by fractured social relationships. This is equally true of rural areas as well as of urban settings. Even though there is a high level of mutual assistance among rural neighbours, especially in times of crisis or emergency, village and country life is also isolating and frequently characterized by petty disputes, parochialism and superficial relationships (Rees, 1950; Williams, 1956; Frankenberg, 1966; Newby, 1979; Bulmer, 1986). Constables on the beat are valued, therefore, not for possible instrumental benefits they may bring in terms of crime prevention but because they represent a desirable social order: stable, regular, constant, predictable, personal, and human.

Public expectations of the police are grounded in a realistic assessment of what can be delivered and do not simply represent an emotional appeal to an imaginary 'golden age' that is now lost. Although there is quite naturally little appreciation that dissensus, crime concern and moral panics represent the *continuities* of social tradition (see Pearson, 1983a, 1989) people realize the intransigent nature of crime in society, and the limited contribution the police can make to its deterrence and resolution. People do not generally have high expectations of the police because they believe them to be handicapped by inadequate resources (which itself can be seen as an ideological construct) and see much crime as incapable of being solved by means that would be tolerable in a liberal democratic society. Whilst for some people these understandings arise out of their experiences with the police, for most people they represent belief-systems founded in 'common sense' untouched by actual contact with police or crime.

## FEAR OF CRIME AND CRIME CONCERN

This set of public evaluations points up a major gulf between police and community understandings of the importance of crime in people's lives. For the police, crime has centrality in constituting people's social relations, blighting the lives of many, instilling fear into most, and distorting the outlook and behaviour of everybody. Given this, it is logical that the 'partnership' approach to policing should focus on crime and that neighbourhood watch itself should be crime-based and crime-oriented. Signs and stickers, property-marking and surveillance exactly express an order of priorities which gives primacy to certain types of crime, its prevention and deterrence. In the official rhetoric, what counts most is cracking crime.

This prioritization of crime is not, however, shared by the public. Crime *is* a feature of the lives of most people, a matter of importance, a matter of concern. It is a factor which is taken into account in all kinds of social decisions: where to live, how to travel to work, where to spend leisure time, when to leave home, when to stay in it, which parts of town to visit, which parts to avoid, which people to associate with and which ones to leave alone. It is built in to evaluations of people, areas and habitats, and incorporated into people's outlooks, perspectives and routines. However, for some, including a majority of women and members of vulnerable ethnic minority groups, crime is more than this, generating fear and instability, narrowing the social space available to them.

For this group, it is important that their fears are constructively addressed and that attempts to delegitimate grounded concerns by 'educating away' fears are resisted. Elderly people frightened by sensationalized media representation of crime, women who are subjected to the imposition of male violence legitimated by the wider culture of masculinity, and ethnic minorities terrorized by persistent racist attacks, all have legitimate fears that need to be addressed and not explained away. This requires, as Ignatieff indicates, concrete and not ideological responses:

> [Progressive politicians] ought to talk less about prisons and policemen and more about rebuilding civic trust among strangers in public places – by giving tenants control over their estates; by creating clubs, bars, gyms and small businesses where kids can create a civic space of their own between the institutions of the home, school and dole office; by creating parks, public monuments and estates which, as the Victorians had the confidence to do, have the kind of beauty and respect for

human scale which demands pride and trust from those who use them.

(Ignatieff, 1983, p. 9)

This in turn feeds into issues relating to property design, the management of public housing and public space, and police delivery systems. Whilst exaggerated claims are often made for the benefits of designing 'defensible space' into public housing (see Newman, 1972; Coleman, 1985; and the observations of Heidensohn, 1989, pp. 27–32), there is widespread agreement that public property can be made less intimidating, more personal and easier to manage. This, of course, locks directly into the political economy which has seen a steady erosion of resources available to local authorities (who, in turn, are bypassed by the structure of NW), undermining their capacity to maintain, improve and manage estates (Audit Commission, 1986). As Bright (1987) points out, extra resources could provide receptionists or door porters in multi-storey blocks, effective door and window security, adequate play and youth facilities, extra street lighting and the like (see, for example, an experiment in the Hilldrop Estate in Islington reported in the *Guardian*, 26 November 1990). Design and management changes of this kind can also be accompanied by a shift in power from local authorities to tenants (Power, 1981, 1988).

For the overwhelming majority of people, however, crime is a subordinate concern. In the lives of ordinary people, other problems predominate: the structural, economic and political problems of housing, employment, transport, and education, and the environmental problems of noise, dirt, pollution, and rubbish. For most people, crime is just one more feature which has to be taken into account, and this is true in both low and high crime areas. As Taub *et al.* point out, although there is a correlation between low crime rates and satisfaction in the neighbourhood, high crime rates do not necessarily have the opposite relationship:

This is not because residents fool themselves and misperceive the fact that crime is a serious problem. . . . Rather, at least below some threshold, crime is viewed as part of a bundle of attributes which determine how one feels toward one's neighborhood. Positive attributes such as property appreciation and an ambience of activity are able to overpower the negative sentiments generated by crime rates. On the other hand, when many elements in the bundle seem to be deteriorating, crime rates take on new significance. They are seen as yet another sign that things are not going well for the neighborhood – property is deteriorating, housing is standing vacant, and perhaps the neighborhood is changing either racially or in its social class composition. Crime rates emphasize one's helplessness in the face of larger negative social processes.

(1981, pp. 117–18)

For most people crime is non-serious and episodic (Gilroy and Sim, 1987) and its material manifestations less significant than its underlying aetiology. There can be no doubt that, at times when there is a crisis of authority in the state operating at the economic, political and ideological level (the 'organic crisis' of Gramsci, 1986, pp. 210–18) and a 'moral panic' is socially and politically constructed (Hall *et al.*, 1978), there may be a widespread and fierce reaction against the 'crime' and 'criminals' said to be responsible for threatening social disorder. When there is no such crisis, however, we found that significant numbers of ordinary people, including many of the property-owning classes, refuse to accord 'crime' and 'criminals' folk-devil status, in some cases because they see crime as a product of the political economy. For the police this is both frustrating and unsettling, as this community beat officer demonstrates:

> I feel as if I am losing my identity as a policeman. I'm entering a sort of grey area. . . . I can't quite adjust to the fact that the car that's sitting on their road, tax out of date, concerns them more than maybe the burglary that occurred a few days ago. They seem to assume that 'OK. We live in a nice house. Sooner or later we're gonna get burgled. But what about this bloody car that's parked outside my house for the last three days? It hasn't moved. Why hasn't something been done about that?'

Equally, it casts grave doubt upon the analysis of the new realist school of criminology which places the victim at the centre of policy planning, and crime as the number one social concern – a matter which we found was not the case even in inner-city areas. It also accounts for the failure of neighbourhood watch to become a true social movement. Neighbourhood watch fails because it is not emergent and does not dovetail into community needs. Legitimate criticisms can be levelled against its failure to address the crimes of the powerful and its encouragement of communities to receive and accept definitions of crime which focus on the powerless (Iadocola, 1985), against its property-owning bias (Donnison *et al.*, 1986; Husain, 1988), and its failure to recognize the home as a source of violence (Russell, 1982; Hanmer and Saunders, 1984; Hall, 1985; Dunhill, 1989), but neighbourhood watch ultimately fails on the ground (instrumentally) because it seeks to elevate the status of crime in people's lives.

## THE VALUE OF SURVEILLANCE INFORMATION

The police were the first, privately, to recognize their failings in this regard. Whatever other motivation lay behind the estab-lishment of schemes at a time when the police as an institution was under intense scrutiny and confronting increasingly powerful calls for greater accountability, the police saw neighbourhood watches as vehicles for increasing the flow of criminal intelligence. They soon discovered, however, that little information of value to them was thereby produced, and that it was almost impossible to hold groups together. This is not a criticism of individual officers, some of whom went to extraordinary lengths to whip up local interest in neighbourhood watch. Rather, it is a comment upon a policing strategy which focused NW on the wrong issue and failed to recognize that even in well-organized communities, as Pearson put it, 'effective communal action is fitful unless organized around a specific grievance such as school closures, road plans etc. and that more usually "community spirit" is represented by only a handful of activists and "busybodies"' (1983b, p. 82). Without public ac-knowledgement of failure, however, the police are trapped into defending the 'success' of neighbourhood watch by inflating the figures of current schemes and making occasional claims to its usefulness in fighting crime. Those areas in which watch schemes have taken root are generally crime-free or low crime areas in terms of police-defined crime. By contrast, in those areas which the police identify with crime, schemes have been difficult or impossible to establish. This split is used in turn to justify police categorizations of society into 'rough' and 'respectable', 'estate' and 'non-estate'. Whilst there is some evidence that people are inhibited from informing because of fear of reprisals (see for example *Guardian*, 15 June 1989: 'Informer fear aids criminals'; Aldridge, 1989, pp. 27–8; Cunningham, 1990), the police are only too eager to stigmatize 'rough' and 'estate' areas as being in the grip of criminals who choke off the flow of intelligence to the police by threatening reprisals against more socially-minded inhabitants.

In contrast to police understandings, there are very many socially valid reasons why the amount of crime information of the kind sought by the police is difficult to increase. In the first place, as some community beat officers acknowledge, most people possess little useful crime-related information. Second, the networks of social control are extraordinarily elaborate, and depend to a large extent upon local histories, traditions and informal systems of control. In recognition of this, some officers in East London, for example, an area associated with an anti-informant tradition, said that they would not encourage people 'to grass' except in respect of 'things like drugs, and child abuse' and similar matters about which there was felt to be broad community consensus favouring crime control strategies. Third, as we have seen in relation to some issues such as 'soft' drugs, paint spraying of walls, and the buying and selling of 'dodgy' merchandise, people may tolerate some level of crime in the interests of living in a pluralist social milieu, where there are few pressures to conform and minimal police interference (cf. Clinard, 1978). It needs to be emphasized, of course, that this conformity also has a gender and racial dimension, involving non-intervention in domestic violence and 'non-grassing up' in respect of racial attacks.

Fourth, 'suspicion', which is the foundation of criminal intelligence, is highly problematic for areas of cultural diversity and heterogenous populations, the main characteristics of inner-city areas. Unlike the police, citizens are generally unwilling to act unless they see conduct which unequivocally refers to criminal behaviour. To encourage citizens to respond to a lower threshold of suspicion invites action based upon 'incongruity' or stereotypical categories, both of which would lend legitimacy to racist constructions employed by the police and fostered by the press. Whilst open to attack on other grounds (Ward, 1984; Gilroy and Sim, 1987; Brogden et al., 1988), the aim of the new realists to enhance the flow of information from the public to the police (Lea and Young, 1984) fails, therefore, because, and contrary to the intentions of new realists themselves, it would transfer racism and bigotry from the private to the public domain, converting it into 'reasonable suspicion'.

Finally, the flow of information to the police will always be restricted by the overriding wish of many people to avoid displacing established relationships in the community. This remains true notwithstanding government attempts to offer substantial rewards (totalling £1 million per annum) to pay people who supply police with information about drugs (see *Guardian*, 15 February 1990). This simply reflects the unresolved contradiction in neighbourhood watch between, on the one hand, the aspiration to create or re-create community solidarity, and, on the other, the encouragement of an informant culture which risks dividing families and turning neighbourhoods against each other (Marx, 1987, 1989).

## CRIME AS AUTHENTIC POLICING

Whatever the difficulties in creating an informant culture, for rank and file officers crime continues to represent authentic policing. Even though crime forms a minor part of their working lives, arrests are infrequent, and much crime is of a mundane, non-serious variety, officers tenaciously cling to a crime-oriented image of police work. This image is used to contradict the value of work connected with serving the community, belittle associated skills involving tact, diplomacy and negotiation, and deride and marginalize community beat officers. It is also invoked to sustain officers during periods of boredom, create group solidarity, and legitimate an aggressive policing style. It additionally expresses the shallow nature of officers' relationships with one another, and this is so notwithstanding the genuine feelings of loyalty and mutual support officers have for one another in times of danger. The tensions and contradictions within the policing mandate, the political nature of policing and the dilemmas this can present, are submerged in a culture which demands *expressions* of commitment, certainty of purpose and worth. As one officer put it,

> Relationships among the relief are extremely superficial. I think what actually leads to stress in the job is the actual relationships among the PCs. It's all superficial. They are so much into their macho image that to obviously discuss such matters with each other would be effeminate and not on: all conversation is very superficial; beer, women and when you're driving along in the car just passing comments about people that are walking past.

The image of authentic policing held by officers finds its fullest expression in the inner cities.

## SUBURBAN AND RURAL POLICING

Before turning to the inner cities, however, we need to reiterate some points about the characteristics of suburban and rural policing. Whilst there are very substantial differences from area to area within forces, as well as between forces, suburban and rural policing overall represent a less intense style of policing: more relaxed, less confrontational, and more favourably received by the inhabitants. The principal complaint from residents is of under-policing, and the consistent call is for an increase in foot patrols and greater visibility of officers. In general, officers appeared more 'in tune' with their local communities. And rural officers were often critical of the behaviour of officers from 'city forces' or 'big forces' (often, in truth, simply 'the Met.') basing their criticism upon press coverage of other forces and 'trade knowledge'. We were constantly urged not to attribute the 'failings' of city forces to officers in rural areas who, it was said, had already had to suffer the 'bureaucracy' of the Police and Criminal Evidence Act 1984, which was 'only really needed to deal with the Met.'. Other officers attributed the problems of city forces to size and expressed concern at recent suggestions favouring forces or even the creation of a national force. Whilst there is some truth in all of this, and a great deal of truth in some of this, many of the characteristics we identify in inner-city policing are present, although in more muted forms, in all the forces we studied, and, in terms of the future of policing, the debates tend to be led by inner-city forces.

## POLICING THE INNER CITY

The inner cities, which themselves constitute the critical sites of policing in terms of the development of police powers and policing styles, classically represent the 'hard' edge of policing. Isolated from the community, both as a consequence of identifiable features of police work such as the shift system but also as a chosen way of dealing with the psychological stress which flows from too close a knowledge of those policed, officers in the inner city adopt an impositional style in which aggression and confrontation are routine components. Even within the inner city, however, this style of policing is not applied to everyone but bears directly upon those sections of the community denigrated in police culture as 'slag' and 'scum', a core part of which in London and Bristol is seen to be the black community.

The search for causal relationships is notoriously difficult and only a partial account is possible. For the police, insofar as they acknowledge the problem, aggressive policing is aberrational rather than routine, an overreaction to the provocative behaviour of 'scum', 'toe-rags', 'scrotes' and 'pukes' (Boesel and Rossi, 1971; Lee, 1981), or the unjustifiable actions of a deviant officer. And it should be remembered, in relation to those officers who locate their own cynicism in the hostile reception they receive from some sections of the community, that every well-intentioned recruit must carry the burden of policing in the same uniform as that worn by all prejudiced or badly-intentioned predecessors. Other officers believe that aggressive policing is not widespread. They see themselves as victims of isolated incidents given currency in the media combined with an uncritical understanding of past practices, as the following Metropolitan Police officer illustrates:

> I think what has changed is that people have become more aware and the press have become more aware of incidents. The classic issue was the assaults on the boys in Holloway, that doesn't help does it? I think, prior to that, a lot of people rightly or wrongly would have read that and thought 'no, impossible', but now that's been proved that it did happen they think it's routine. At the end of the day people have got to understand that in a force of 27,000 you are going to have bad ones, but in the past you did as well although they wouldn't believe a policeman would do any wrong. They wouldn't believe that a policeman would steal, and they wouldn't believe that a policeman would beat someone up for no reason. When you see that in North Wales where they had beaten someone to the ground, or a policeman convicted for theft, they see that and suddenly they realise that you do get bad policemen. I think some people don't hold us in quite the esteem that they used to, albeit that it's more of a sensible viewpoint because you can't accept that every policeman is good.

Whilst there may be some truth in this view, our research demonstrates the essentially coercive nature of inner-city policing. Police negative categorizations of citizens are not merely private typologies used to position individuals within the relief group or reinforce police subculture. Rather, they have been internalized to constitute a policing *ideology* which informs and directs operational practice. Although it is true that many police encounters with citizens who rank low in police esteem are unremarkable, even friendly, there is ample evidence, from citizens and police alike, of the routine use of aggressive tactics against certain groups in society, especially members of ethnic minorities. The evidence of our research supports the observations of Foster (1989) that the bad reputation of whole police stations has a firm foundation in reality.

Individuals are stopped and searched *because* they are black or *because* they possess one of the other attributes which qualify them as 'slag' in the eyes of the police. When walking along the street or when stopped by an officer, the citizen may be subjected to various kinds of provocation, which may range from the overt use of derogatory epithets to, as one officer told us, the use of feigned subservience. ('Just calling them "Sir" in the right way can upset them.') The process of 'winding up' the citizen is designed to produce a negative reaction which can then be used to legitimate a 'tough' response. The key to this, as one officer told us, is to transform the situation so that the officer's behaviour toward the citizen is subordinated to the (presumptively unjustifiable) response of the citizen to the officer:

> Basically you react to how people react to you, and so to a certain extent your interest in them is based on how they react to you reacting to them. A lot of policemen get a little bit annoyed because more people don't run away, because then you know you have got something if they run away.

This peremptory and impositional style of policing requires substantial social distance between officers and citizens, thus giving a further push to the isolation of the police associated with their claims to professionalism.

This position of the police in relation to citizens is held in place by an entrenched occupational culture which celebrates rank and file monopoly of insider knowledge of crime and criminals. From the perspective of the rank and file, management is seen to be involved in the separate function of legitimating policing by systematically denying ground level realities. This is given further credence by the view that senior officers are not in touch with day-to-day policing practices and by their willingness to 'betray' the rank and file by occasionally sacrificing officers – 'real officers, doing real police work' – through disciplinary mechanisms in order to placate the public.

This in turn is simply evidence of a basic contradiction within the police mandate. That contradiction is not principally concerned with the *means* of policing but with its *ends* (Balbus, 1973; Rumbaut and Bittner, 1979). Essentially this involves a tension between the police as a service-oriented body and the police as the agency for order-maintenance. This tension is not accidental or new but goes back to the formation of the modern police force in the nineteenth century. Whilst the first British police were public-order police (Bowden, 1978), police reformers, such as Chadwick, fostered the service role precisely to legitimate more coercive functions. Thus, Chadwick argued that it would

> exercise a beneficial influence on the labouring classes . . . by showing them that they are cared for by the authorities, and are not, as they must but too commonly suppose, merely and exclusively the subjects of coercion.
>
> (Donajgrodski, 1977, p. 67, cited by Reiner, 1985, p. 57)

The services performed in the nineteenth century, such as inspecting bridges and waking people up, were seen at the time by rank and file officers as 'extraneous' duties, not part of their core mandate (Steedman, 1984). Parallel sentiments towards 'service' duties are clearly felt by their modern counterparts.

The contradiction in the police mandate helps make sense of police internal structures as well as of the differential experiences citizens have of policing. Thus the division between community beat officers and relief officers encapsulates the division between the expressive ideological function of the police and its repressive or instrumental purpose. It leads to schisms within apparently homogenous groups (such as relief) and legitimates 'resistance' by officers opposed to occupational cultures. It also accounts for the endemic contradictions between the universalistic claims made for policing – equal treatment for all – and its uneven and sectional practices (Norrie and Adelman, 1988). Neighbourhood watch, in turn, confronts the service model of policing and reveals it as a myth.

The inherent contradiction between 'community' and 'fire-brigade' policing is well brought out in the views that residents have of the police in inner cities, as in the following examples:

*Avon and Somerset resident*

I know they try and go into schools and that, so that if they have a good relationship with the kids in schools they will grow up OK – but it doesn't work like that because the young ones have brothers and sisters and parents that they see being ill treated by the same policemen who are coming and purportedly being friends. So it doesn't work in this area. It's like a way forward in other areas to get the police in the schools. But I don't think it works round here. . . . I think sometimes the kids are a bit mixed up because the policeman will come in and he will be OK, but if you are on the street with a couple of your big brothers or whatever you will stand there and watch them being hassled or whatever. So you are getting two pictures sent to you and it makes them confused.

*Metropolitan resident*

I would like to see the bobby on the beat, without any arms, and who does not deal in civil disturbances, who does his job as a policeman keeping the law. I wouldn't like that same bobby being involved in riot control at all. I would prefer to have a paramilitary force, like they have in Europe. So when you see people being bashed over the head with a truncheon you know it's the paramilitary riot police, and not the policeman on the beat, because after seeing him hit people over the head, it kind of jaundices your attitude to the ordinary bobby on the beat. Your attitude is wary and not trustful. In this country it's one and the same person, and it must therefore colour his attitude, it must affect him as a person, having to do those jobs which I don't think he should do. That should be for another force, a riot police force. You can hate them and never come into contact with them, unless, of course, you're throwing pebbles at them.

It was also apparent in the views of those few officers who reported themselves as disturbed by developments within policing that they saw as contradicting expressed commitments to community policing. The following Avon and Somerset CBO, for example, was critical of the trend towards para-military policing and the under-investment in community policing initiatives. He sought to explain this trend in terms of the urban–rural divide:

Well you have to understand that in any area of any force, you have the rural and the city area and policy will be dictated by how those areas are. We are inner city so perhaps I cannot expect much emphasis to be placed on community policemen. It ought to be, I think it ought to be. But they are spending more money on riot gear, making sure police have spent more money on a new sort of armour bus and of course their community aspect is of a lower priority whereas perhaps in the more rural areas, because all you have is community policing in cars, they have a higher priority.

Whilst services continue to be performed by the police and play a substantial part in day-to-day policing (Banton, 1964; Cumming *et al.*, 1965), these tasks are carried out as a by-product of their availability and their possession of coercive powers (Bittner, 1967; Reiner, 1985) and not, in the main, as part of a voluntarily chosen mandate. When police are called upon to undertake service as an *objective* of policing, their claims to respond to needs defined by the community look to the observer like mere ideological window dressing (Brogden, 1982). Just as the expressive arm of policing was originally needed to enable the police to penetrate the counterveiling norms of the 'roughs' (Cohen, P., 1979), neighbourhood watch is not discharged for any intrinsic value it might have but for instrumental benefits (gaining intelligence, observation posts and the like) it *might* bring for the police (Bridges and Bunyan, 1983; Gordon, 1984). Seen in this way expressive and repressive forms of policing are not contradictory; rather, repressive policing demands 'knowledge' of the community and penetration of the community by means of expressive forms, including neighbourhood watch. This gives substance to the analysis of Bridges (1981) who has argued that, in its ideal form

> community policing merges at the local level the coercive and consensual functions of government, enabling the police to wield a frightening mixture of repressive powers, on the one hand, and programmes of social intervention, on the other, as mutually reinforcing tools in their efforts to control . . . black and working class communities.

This essential dichotomy within the police would be much more difficult to sustain if policing was simply a site for contradictory practices. It is much more than this: it is a site for contradictory *lawful* practices. Different styles, forms and delivery systems of policing operate and flourish within an overarching legal structure which is permissive. This operates both at the macro-legal level in terms of the very foundations of police authority – constabulary autonomy and constabulary independence – and at the micro-legal level where individual laws and sets of rules act not as restraints on the police but resources for them (McBarnet, 1981; McConville *et al.*, 1991). It is the law, therefore, which provides the political space within which a distinctive occupational culture can flourish.

## SYMBOLIC LOCATIONS

The style of policing which this occupational culture expresses is uniquely focused in police-defined 'symbolic locations'. Whilst inner-city streets, through their use as the main leisure areas for poor working-class youths freed from the ties of the family and school but short of cash (Brogden *et al.*, 1988, p. 148), have always been important sites for the reproduction of social order, the weight of policing and the crucible of policing policy is most closely connected to those areas identified by the police as 'symbolic locations'. For London, these were defined by Sir Kenneth Newman, then Commissioner of the Metropolitan Police, in the following terms:

> Throughout London there are locations where unemployed youth – often black youths – congregate; where the sale and purchase of drugs, the exchange of stolen property and illegal drinking and gaming is not uncommon. The youths regard these locations as their territory. Police are viewed as intruders, the symbol of authority – largely white authority – in a society that is responsible for all their grievances about unemployment, prejudice and discrimination. They closely equate with the criminal 'rookeries' of Dickensian London.
>
> (cited in Gilroy and Sim, 1987, at p. 100)

Symbolic locations of this character fell within our research sites in both London and Bristol and were viewed in these terms by rank and file officers to whom we spoke. Whilst this police construction of symbolic locations reinforces authoritarian policing styles and constitutes a demand for extra police powers so long as these areas are said to be immune from 'standard' policing expectations, there is an apparent dispute as to the operational implications that flow from this police analysis.

On the one hand, some argue that 'conventional' policing is suspended in these locations which thereby become 'no-go' areas. This approach is exemplified by Graef in his ethnographic account of British police officers. According to Graef, the police engage in 'soft' policing in 'sensitive areas', which accordingly become sanitized zones in which 'embargoes are placed on conventional arrests, on movements in and out of the area by other police officers and on the handling of controversial figures in the community' (1989, p. 102). Various officers in Graef's account describe how they were 'warned-off' by senior officers, and how they were required to adopt 'softly, softly' strategies, as in the following examples:

An officer in a sensitive area explained that the police 'don't go trying to arrest people unless it is something bad. If we know who they are we just go round sometime during the night . . . and ask them to come with us. His friends are not around so we can avoid disorder.'

(Graef, 1989, p. 106)

'Police units were not allowed to respond to anything that was happening around the All Saints Road in case it inflamed our relationships with the people in the road.'

(ibid., p. 113)

'If we go out somewhere to do a raid, if we want to go through that subdivision's patch, we have to ask permission first. It's usually denied, so we have to go round it. It's like the Berlin Wall.'

(ibid., p.107)

The implication is clear that, whatever the original intention of Newman in identifying symbolic locations, the police have learned that 'normal' policing invites resistance and, in order to avoid disorder, have 'gone soft' in these areas (see the discussion of policing in Toxteth, Liverpool in *R. v. Oxford ex parte Levey, The Independent*, 30 October 1986). In this scenario, black people get *preferential* treatment.

A different picture comes out of the Institute of Race Relations. Continuing the tradition laid down by Joe Hunte (1966) in his pamphlet, *Nigger Hunting in England*, the Institute of Race

Relations argues that there has been over-policing of suspected black offences and of black events, and underpolicing of black victimization. The institute argues that, throughout the 1970s, the police practised a consistent pattern of over-policing black events, a pattern which intensified in the 1980s with raids, saturation policing, widespread stops and searches, routine patrolling of inner-city areas with riot squads, all underpinned by continuous intelligence-gathering and surveillance. The strategy shifted in the 1980s from 'law-and-order' policing to 'public order' policing, with the focus on inner-city symbolic locations: estates, clubs, and political and cultural meeting places. In the institute's view, this strategy had a much wider impact on the black community, with the police cultivating the press in order to gain support for their policies and to stigmatize the black community, as by dramatizing the issue of 'black street crime' in an effort to discredit the Scarman report on the Brixton disorders. The allegations that black areas are given preferential policing and that some are even 'no-go' areas is seen in different terms:

> Such stories frequently appear in advance of, or directly follow-
> ing, large-scale police raids against black community
> institutions and meeting places. In effect, they serve to justify
> such operations and support police demands for additional
> powers and resources.
>
> (Institute of Race Relations, 1987, at p. 53)

This would help explain, according to the Institute, the way in which the press often seeks to stigmatize whole areas or estates as criminogenic, as in the characterization of such places as the Stockwell Park and Broadwater Farm estates in London. In addition to all this, the police, it is said, do not do enough to protect black people from racist attacks and tend to criminalize those who fight against their racist attackers. This is achieved by playing down the significance of racist attacks; redefining these as street issues, hooliganism, or neighbouring disputes; and blaming the victim, such as, by saying that the incidents were family feuds, committed for financial gain, or self-inflicted. In this account, therefore, black people, far from getting preferential policing, suffer from discriminatory and *differential* policing.

In our view, there is no essential contradiction between these two accounts. Policing of symbolic locations is characterized by a mixture of preferential and differential policing strategies which creates both a deep sense of outrage in the community and confusion in the minds of rank and file officers. For residents, the temper of policing is set by the routinely unsympathetic character of day-to-day policing and dramatized by those occasions on which the police utilize heavy-handed, saturation, or repressive methods. For the police, periods of relative inactivity in the face of open infractions of law manifest an unwillingness on the part of the force to 'deal with' the problem and an abdication of the principles of equal enforcement. To the observer, the contradiction between the claims to equal enforcement and the order maintenance function of the police results in a style of policing which is arbitrary and lacking in empathy.

In these symbolic locations, as was the case with the slum areas of Victorian cities (Davis, 1989), there is an observable element of what police officers see as 'preferential' treatment. Rank and file officers, as we have seen, are under instructions not to clamp cars in certain areas or engage in 'process chases'. When an incident arises on the street, officers may be instructed to withdraw even where they see offences being committed. One Avon and Somerset officer told us, for example, of an incident which turned into a 'mini-riot' during which some 'kids' set fire to an abandoned car. The rank and file wanted to give chase and arrest the kids but they were 'told to retreat'. Other officers recounted similar stories and told us that these strategies were particularly favoured by 'butterfly officers' who were at stations for short periods of time and were determined to avoid any 'flare ups' which could suggest an inability to direct and manage. For relief officers in particular, strategies of these kinds collectively amounted to the abandonment of policing even though, of course, full enforcement of the law is not contemplated by the police in *any* area of the country.

At the same time, in public pronouncements about force policy senior officers offer these localities 'community policing'. This is intended, in the rhetoric of senior officers, to complement 'soft policing' by reliefs and to strengthen police–citizen relations. Community officers we spoke to, however, told us that they had little or nothing to do with residents. Often working in pairs in 'sensitive' areas, officers had little interaction with the community and, many told us, this was exactly how they liked to police. An officer in Avon and Somerset who was critical of this style of policing precisely because there was no attempt to integrate with the community pinpointed the operational shortcomings of this system in these terms:

> In those areas the officers are not being community officers. They will go down there, walk around, not speak to anyone, and come back again. Totally morale destroying as such. I done it for six months and hated it because I wanted to get involved with people, and I wasn't given the back up to do it. There is a community down there, it's just that you have to deal with it very sensitively. But the fact that I am walking around with a 6'6" police officer who wants to go around arresting people makes my life very difficult if I want to stop and chat to someone. The way he wants to carry on going, of course, what with you policing in twos which is necessary in that area, it's impossible to be a community officer when you work in pairs. Very difficult especially if the other officer that you are working with doesn't think the same way you do.

There is thus no real attempt at an operational level to negotiate an acceptable policing presence with the community, many of whose members have a negative, even hostile, view of the police.

The maintenance of this negative view of policing has to be understood against the backcloth of another continuity in police strategies associated with 'repressive' policing, rather than in terms of the ineffectiveness of the half-hearted 'community policing' described above. Although forces sometimes use beat officers to walk through communities, these symbolic locations remain the sites for 'heavy' policing methods: saturation of the area with officers, the use of patrol vans to provide an intimidating presence, and police raids on venues important to the local community. The threat of community resistance and street disorders may reduce the frequency of such highly organized (that is, institutionalized) raids and tactics but do not lead to their abandonment. Equally, the perceived threat of resistance to the police reinforces the 'heavy-handedness' of day-to-day policing, which continues to be driven by typologies based on 'incongruities': being young and hanging around street corners, being black and driving an expensive car, being young and male on the street late at night, being a woman and stepping out of line, being black and being 'out of area' (see for example Policy Studies Institute, 1983; Brogden, 1985; Tchaikovsky, 1989). And in undertaking routine practices, officers may vent any resentment they have about being 'restrained' by senior officers, goading citizens into aggressive responses, using unnecessary force, or going in 'mob-handed'.

Indeed, if resistance is anticipated then individual officers will on their own initiative (rather than as a result of any orders from above) avoid routine contact with the citizen and also the 'ordinary arrest'. Every contact will be seen as having a potential for confrontation, every arrest a potential for violence and disorder, and will only be approached by the police on relief in, and with, maximum force. Despite the protests of rank and file officers against the supposed 'soft' community policing of black areas, there is an essential congruity between policing policies toward 'symbolic locations' and the day-to-day policing practices of officers on the beat in these areas. Both are based on the need for exceptional and therefore discriminatory policing of the black community.

The result, so far as residents are concerned, is a style of policing which is contingent and arbitrary. In a heightened form, the relationship between police and the black community mirrors accounts of police relationships with the 'rough' white working-class communities described by Phil Cohen (1979) and Mike Brogden (1982). Cohen, in describing the transformation of policing in Islington over the period 1875–1935 cites oral testimony of an Islington resident describing police brutality in the street and comments, 'The sense of shock registered is not then at the actual violence metered out. This is accepted as a normal feature of relations between adult authority and youth. *What does hurt is the sudden and arbitrary nature of its occurrence.*' (Cohen, P., 1979, at p. 123, emphasis added). Brogden, in describing similar conflict between sections of the working class and the police states, 'For the . . . participants in the street economy . . . attitudes to the police institution throughout the first century of policing remained essentially unchanged. They were subject to *continuing, occasional,* and *apparently "arbitrary" culls*' (1982, at pp. 180–1, emphasis added). Rather than being 'no-go' areas, symbolic locations are better understood as 'stop-go' areas. It is thus perfectly possible for the police to hold the view that black areas are given preferential treatment, because they interpret the moments when coercive policing is suspended as constituting its abandonment. At the same time, while residents in these areas may believe that they are continuously subject to coercive policing because they see occasional but continuing raids as symptomatic of standard repression, other sections of the public may think that policing has been abandoned in these areas, thus allowing residents to get away with crime.

The sense that residents have of policing in these areas is, however, constituted by and finds expression in routine encounters as well as in set-piece battles and reactions to heavy-handed raids. The muttered comments of police officers, their sarcastic and confrontational methods of speaking to residents, matched by the reciprocal behaviour of residents in terms of 'blanking out' of officers, teeth-sucking, and the shouting of abuse, both symbolize and reproduce embittered relationships. We agree with Foster (1989) that it is a mistake to underestimate the fears officers have about the challenge black people pose to their authority. In both Avon and Somerset and the Metropolitan Police, we found, as had Foster, that officers experienced a strong undercurrent of threat and unpredictability which led some to walk down 'the front line in order to assert their territorial right of way' (Foster, 1989, p. 144). We also found that some officers avoided 'flashpoint' areas for similar reasons: as one Avon and Somerset officer said in relation to a road in a 'sensitive' area of the city, 'I cannot see the point of walking down there because all you get is a load of abuse hurled at you and all you're doing is losing face.' The relationships are all the more hostile because the essential dispute is less about law and order and more about the resistance of the community and the police demand for deference. In their refusal to adopt a submissive attitude, black people classically present the most powerful modern challenge to imposed police authority. As Sir Kenneth Newman (cited in Gilroy and Sim, 1987, p. 100) put it when discussing the 'symbolic locations',

> If allowed to continue, locations with these characteristics assume symbolic importance – a negative symbolism of the inability of the police to maintain order. Their existence encourages law breaking elsewhere, affects public perceptions of police effectiveness, heightens fear of crime and reinforces the phenomenon of urban decay.

Thus, as Gilroy and Sim point out, police concern is primarily at the symbolic level at which these localities attract police wrath, because of 'their capacity to convey the limitations of police power and to signify the fragility of the order which the police are able to impose' (1987, p. 100). The police construction of these symbolic locations is used both to legitimate police methods for dealing with the communities themselves and to justify claims for additional para-military powers for more general use. They are another indication of the rise of the strong state (Centre for Contemporary Cultural Studies, 1982; Sim, 1990).

All this points to a central problem which has tended to become marginalized by left realists and underplayed by the victimization movement; namely, *that there is a core problem with the police*. It is not necessary to go to the critics of the police to see this; it is firmly embedded in the way that officers see their role and conceptualize their mission. In the critical inner-city locations, and to a lesser extent elsewhere, officers see themselves as estranged from local communities and heavily dependent upon a few individuals to provide them with points of contact and thus the semblance of 'policing by consent'. Nowhere is this better characterized than in the way officers talk about police stations.

In inner-city areas, police stations are in fact the true 'symbolic locations'. It is in the police station that is housed the base of 'important' knowledge of the community in the form of the collator's office; it is the centre for the creation and celebration of group culture; it is the site in which officers can re-make and re-tell their own policing histories; and it provides the base from which officers go out to police the community and to which they repeatedly return to re-confirm their own identities. The centrality of the station appears in the following quotations from officers:

*Metropolitan community beat officer*
There is an institution at the moment that, if you are on early turn which is six in the morning to two in the afternoon, at eight o'clock everyone has to have tea together. Now, if you think 'I'll go out and do my jobs' because you are enjoying yourself out there doing that job, talking to people, shopkeepers, stallholders or whatever, if you don't come back for your tea, you are not fitting in and people will say 'Well where is he? Is he alright?'. And rather than going out as individuals for eight hours, interacting and mixing with the community and, you know, finishing your work and going home for the day, there's pressure on you to do precisely the reverse because if you don't come into the station you know that they'll think you're unsociable. If you disappear, you know, really disappear, like into the community and get lost for eight hours, they are wondering

not where you are, you know, not whether you've disappeared and are maybe skiving off, but if you're not there, so that people can see you, at the station, and you're not coming back for your cup of tea and stuff, you're *unsociable*. It really is like that. (original emphasis)

*Avon and Somerset community beat officer*
Relief officers often engage in backstabbing. When you're out of the room they'll do that – 'He's not very popular because he doesn't usually come in for rests, he'll stay out so you won't see him for eight hours.'

*Avon and Somerset community beat officer*
I'm criticized for all sorts of things: I am out there having cups of tea all the time with women . . . again, the fact that I take my cup of tea on my beat and don't come back to the station.

Police stations thus represent more than police territory: they symbolize the militaristic and colonialistic nature of inner-city policing, the garrison mentality of officers who are banded together around a common occupational culture, and the social and political distance that is maintained between the police and the public. In this context, it is necessary to remember that whilst neighbourhood watch may be a failure in instrumental terms, it continues to have an important ideological function in depicting the police as a 'listening force' and in representing them as community-based.

This must not be understood as an argument for laying all the problems of society at the door of the police. On the contrary, the central problems remain the political and economic sectionaliza-tion of the population, patriarchy and racism. Nevertheless, it remains true that the police reproduce this fractured social order in extreme forms, help stigmatize whole groups as beyond the pale of accredited society, politicize their own prejudices through law and order debates, and lend legitimacy to more repressive forms of policing. The independence of police culture, its low visibility, as well as its operation at the 'front line' of policing supports Foucault's (1979) analysis that social control is no longer imposed from above and outside the fabric of social life by a sovereign person; 'rather, it is embedded in the very structure of social relations themselves' (Shearing, 1981a, p. 293) – but still legitim-ated by the state. Watching neighbours may provide an interesting pastime; watching the police is a political imperative.

# Appendix

The research on which this study is based was carried out in three police areas of England and Wales chosen for their different policing problems and for their varied policies towards neighbourhood watch (NW). The Avon and Somerset Force could justifiably claim, with the Kingsdown Neighbourhood Watch project in Bristol started in February 1983, to have inaugurated the first complete NW project in Britain. Since that date the force has continued to support NW although, after actively marketing schemes in the early years, it now relies upon public initiation. Even if it was not the pioneer of NW, the Metropolitan Police Force can claim to be the one that gave NW its greatest impetus, with Sir Kenneth Newman making NW a central part of his new policing strategy launched in September 1983. Like Avon and Somerset, the Metropolitan Police revised their early policy and now rely upon public initiation for new schemes. Our third force, Gwent Constabulary, has taken a much less prominent role in NW, force policy being confined to providing official support to schemes initiated by the public but without official advertising and other forms of encouragement or promotion.

In addition to their stance on NW, the three forces provided us with a wide range of policing problems and policing styles. The Metropolitan Police District, with some 28,500 officers, covers a wide spectrum of suburban and inner-city areas, with some of the most prominent political locations in the policing debates and notorious problems in the area of police–ethnic minority relations. Avon and Somerset, with over 3,000 officers, also offers a wide mix of policing problems with parts of the Brisol area having gained national prominence in the street disorders of 1980. The third force, Gwent, is comparatively small in policing terms, with approximately 1,000 officers, and few of the inner-city problems confronting the other two forces, but having its own problems in covering a scattered rural population.

So far as the police are concerned, our main source of data collection, supplemented by limited observational work, is derived from in-depth interviews conducted with individual officers. Problems with taping, such as excessive background noise, reduced the number of usable police interviews to 206. With the consent of officers involved, interviews were tape-recorded under conditions which guaranteed the anonymity and confidentiality of all police personnel. Steps have been taken in the text, using standard socio-legal techniques, to ensure these research conditions are met and that no individual officer can be identified from the interview extracts which we print. Only one officer in all three forces approached did not consent to be tape-recorded.

The sub-divisions in which the research was located were chosen in conjunction with each police force. Each force was concerned to ensure that we had a free choice as to location, subject to securing a broad cross-section of areas and, in one case, to avoiding some sites in which other research was current. In all cases, the police were scrupulously fair in avoiding influencing the course of the research and in giving us freedom to select our research sites. In the Metropolitan Police District, interviews were conducted with officers located in five sub-divisional areas, two of which were inner-city, two suburban, and one mixed urban and suburban. In Avon and Somerset, three sub-divisional areas were covered, one inner-city, one suburban, and one rural. Finally, in Gwent interviews were conducted with officers from two city sub-divisions, and from a range of other sites covering villages and towns.

In each research site, we attempted to interview all available community beat officers (described variously in different forces as home beat officers, residential beat officers, permanent beat officers, sectional officers, and village police officers) because these officers have special responsibility amongst other duties for supporting NW schemes. Each interview lasted for approximately one hour and involved asking officers questions about how they came to be involved in community beat work, the morale and status of community beat officers, the kinds of work they undertook, the problems they encountered, their involvement in neighbourhood watch, their relationship with relief officers and with supervisors and senior officers, and their future career plans. Using a semi-structured interview schedule, all questions were non-directed in nature (for example, How did you come to be a community beat officer? What do you think is the status of a community beat officer in this force? What, if any, are the problems on your beat in policing terms?) with supplementary questions dependent upon the responses of each officer.

Since community beat officers are drawn from and interact with the uniform relief we also sought a parallel sample of interviews with relief officers in each research site. As with community beat officers, interviews with the uniformed reliefs were based upon non-directed questions, tape-recorded, and lasted on average about the same time as interviews with community beats. Officers were asked about the advantages and disadvantages of relief work, whether they would consider applying for a community beat posting, their working relationships with community beat officers, the kinds of work they undertook, the problems they encountered, their understanding of NW, and their relationships with supervisory officers.

In respect of both sets of officer, we sought a broad spread in terms of age, length of police service, gender and race. In all these respects we were successful except in terms of race, our samples consisting almost entirely of white officers. This outcome was not in any way influenced by the particular forces with whom research access was negotiated but simply reflects the low numbers of officers from ethnic minority backgrounds in the police as a whole.

In each of the research sites we also undertook surveys of residents, employing a systematic household sample stratified according to both socio-economic status and level of neighbourhood watch involvement, and including areas where schemes had not been established. In total, interviews were conducted with 229 residents. Our intention was to conduct a one in six interview sample but, because of resource problems, we were forced to concentrate on small sites covering 60 to 100 houses. One consequence of this is a bias in favour of neighbourhood watch, which tends to be less successful in larger sites unless supported by a very substantial administrative network of the kind not usually apparent. Nevertheless England and Wales are noteworthy for their relatively large (compared with the US) neighbourhood watch schemes (Bennett, 1990, p. 20) with at least one reported to cover over 3,000 households (Trotman et al., 1984). Although, therefore, our sample may be in this respect atypical, with an overemphasis on smaller schemes, the bias should tend to exaggerate the successful elements of NW rather than to expose its weaknesses. The basis of the survey in the household (as against in individuals) meant also a bias in favour of older sections of the population, which was mitigated to some extent by requesting, in a range of cases, an interview with younger (but over the age of 16) members of the household unit.

The sites chosen for the survey of residents covered households with a broad range of socio-economic characteristics, as described below:

*Sites   Neighbourhood watch areas*

1    An inner-city area with a multi-racial population living in terraced accommodation, some unmodernized, some converted into multi-lets, and some modernized

2    An affluent suburban street of large semi-detached houses built in the 1920s, occupied exclusively by white families

3    An area of affluent suburban residences, mostly detached, occupied by owner-occupier white families

4    A road which combines council houses, rented accommodation, and owner-occupied houses, exclusively white

5    Affluent suburban semi-detached property owned by white families

6    A village in a rural setting dominated by owner-occupied detached houses owned by well-off white families and retired individuals

7    A multi-racial area of poor quality older terraced housing, some council-owned, occupied by low income working-class families

8    A white area of good quality semi-detached housing with some properties converted for multi-lets

9    An area of Victorian terraced housing with a mixture of elderly residents, young affluent first-time buyers, and low income working-class people, all of whom are white

10    A multi-racial area of good quality semi-detached housing with some properties converted to multi-lets

11    A multi-racial area with a very mixed housing stock includ-

ing run-down council estates and gentrified terraced property

12    A white affluent suburban area with detached and semi-detached houses occupied by families

*Sites*   *Non-neighbourhood watch areas*

1    A multi-racial area of terraced housing, some council-owned, occupied by both low-income families and better-off individuals

2    A council estate for white elderly people based upon dividing up large houses into good-quality flats

3    A multiracial area with a mixed housing stock a lot of which are owner-occupied, but including some council property and some rented and bed-sit accommodation

4    A mostly white area of unimproved terraced housing with a lot of old people and low-income families

5    A run-down, inner-city council estate with a multiracial population

6    A multiracial area of large terraced housing much of which is split into flats

7    A white area of good-quality semi-detached housing with a few properties converted for multi-lets

8    A multiracial area of working-class people in a mixture of terraced, council and multi-occupancy accommodation

9    A white rural village with a mixture of council property, rented and owner-occupied accommodation occupied by low-income families

10   A predominantly white area of good-quality housing including semi-detached and multi-let properties, with a few council houses

Each household was initially approached by means of a standard letter which explained the identity of the researcher, a system by which this could be verified by those who were concerned over the bona fides of the research, and the broad nature of the inquiry as involving crime in the locality. The letter explained that the researcher would return a few days later at a fixed time and date, and that the interview would be anonymous and confidential.

Where, as happened in a few cases, repeated visits had failed to locate anyone at the selected address, the property was vacant or had been demolished, the household next door was then approached. When residents were seen directly, the question of tape-recording the interview was raised. In six cases, the request to tape-record was refused. In all cases we tried to ensure that no other household member was present at the interview but this sometimes proved impossible to secure. One likely consequence of this was that it would reduce the occasions on which a victim of violence or other abuse within the household would indicate that the household was not a safe haven.

All respondents were initially asked questions about their general feelings toward and ties to their neighbourhood (for example, Do you consider yourself to be part of a neighbourhood? Is the area a neighbourhood in any way? Is it a distinctive area? Is it an area where people help each other or where they mainly go their own way? Is there a community here? Do you feel part of a community?). Residents were then asked non-directed questions designed to tease out their views about problems in the area and the importance of crime and fear of crime in their lives (for example, What, if any, are the problems for you in this area? What about in other areas? Would you say that there is a crime problem in this area? If so, what is the nature of that problem? If so, in what way would you say it is serious? Is the crime problem something that concerns you in particular?) Questions were also put about their understandings of suspiciousness (for example, What sort of person, if any, would arouse your suspicions in this area? What sort of behaviour, if any, would arouse your suspicions in this area? What, if anything, would you do if you saw something suspicious?) and of their general evaluation of the local police (for example, Are you satisfied with your local police? Taking everything into account, would you say that the police in the area do a good job or a bad job?).

In all areas residents were asked questions about their knowledge of and attitudes toward neighbourhood watch (for example, Do you know what neighbourhood watch is? What do you think neighbourhood watch is supposed to achieve? Do you think neighbourhood watch is a good idea? What are its advantages or disadvantages? ). In scheme areas, residents were asked whether they were members of the scheme, their reasons for joining or not joining, and the effects, if any, the scheme had on such matters as personal or household security, crime rates, and relationships with the neighbours and the police. Members were asked about their involvement in the scheme. Non-members were asked whether they would be willing to be involved in neighbourhood watch if a scheme were set up in their area.

As with all surveys, this piece of research is subject to a number of technical limitations, some of the more important of which need to be mentioned here. In the first place, the research, based as it is upon samples, faces problems of representativeness. So far as the police are concerned, whilst the selected forces covered a variety of policing problems clearly only three of the forty-three forces in England and Wales were included. Moreover, although some officers with supervisory responsibilities were interviewed, the research did not attempt to obtain a systematic management perspective. So far as residents are concerned, the basis of the research in NW created an inevitable bias in favour of the propertied classes, and the choice of the household as the basic survey unit tended to cause a lack of representativeness amongst the younger population (who tend to be out when daytime and evening interviews are conducted!). A second limitation is the relative lack of attention given to crime *within* households committed by one unit-member against another. The focus on neighbourhood watch inevitably concentrates attention on external (public) crime and the current research has, therefore, little contribution to make to important debates about family violence and the like. A third limitation, which applies only to some parts of the interview material, is the reliance upon judgements made by respondents who may well employ different definitions. Thus, for example, whilst one individual may express 'satisfaction' with the job done by the police even where they have failed to solve a crime of which the respondent was the victim, another may express 'dissatisfaction' precisely because of such a failure. The problems of comparability of this kind are endemic to all such surveys, and can be mitigated only, as here, by extensive extracts from respondents' answers to show their fuller reasoning. Wherever possible we made a concerted attempt in selecting quotations to ensure that published extracts are representative of the different groups of respondents encountered in the research.

# Bibliography

Alderson, J. (1979) *Policing Freedom*, Plymouth: Macdonald and Evans.
Aldridge, R. (1989) *Neighbourhood Watch: The Experience of Four Schemes*, London: Home Office Crime Prevention Unit.
Alex, N. (1976) *New York Cops Talk Back*, New York: Wiley.
Anderton, K. (1985) *The Effectiveness of Home Watch Schemes in Cheshire*, Chester: Cheshire Constabulary.
Audit Commission (1986) *Managing the Crisis in Council Housing*, London: HMSO.
Bains, S. (1989) 'Crimes against women', in C. Dunhill (ed.), *The Boys in Blue*, London: Virago.
Balbus, I. (1973) *Dialectics of Legal Repression*, Beverly Hills, Calif.: Russell Sage Foundation.
Baldwin, R. and Kinsey, R. (1982) *Police Powers and Politics*, London: Quartet Books.
Banton, M. (1964) *The Policeman in the Community*, London: Tavistock.
—— (1973) *Police-Community Relations*, London: Collins.
Bayley, D. and Mendelsohn, H. (1968) *Minorities and the Police*, New York: Free Press.
Bennett, T. (1979) 'The social distribution of criminal labels', *British Journal of Criminology* 19: 134.
—— (1989) 'The neighbourhood watch experiment', in R. Morgan and D. Smith (eds), *Coming to Terms with Policing*, London: Routledge.
—— (1990) *Evaluating Neighbourhood Watch*, Aldershot: Gower.
Bennett, T. and Wright, R. (1984) *Burglars on Burglary: Prevention and the Offender*, Aldershot: Gower.
Bent, A. (1974) *The Politics of Law Enforcement*, Toronto: Lexington.
Benyon, J. (1984) 'The policing issues', in J. Benyon (ed.), *Scarman and After*, Oxford: Pergamon Press.
—— (1986) *A Tale of Failure: Race and Policing*, Policy Papers in Ethnic Relations No. 3, Warwick: University of Warwick.
Bittner, E. (1967) 'The police on skid row: a study in peacekeeping', *American Sociological Review* 32: 699.
—— (1970) *The Functions of Police in Modern Society*, Chevy Chase, Md.: National Institute of Mental Health.

Black, D. (1970) 'Production of crime rates', *American Sociological Review* 35: 733.

—— (1972) 'The social organisation of arrest', *Stanford Law Review* 23: 1087.

Black, D. and Reiss, A. (1967) 'Patterns of behaviour in police and citizen transactions', in vol. 2(1) *Studies in Crime and Law Enforcement in Major Metropolitan Areas*, Washington DC: US Government Printing Office.

Blom-Cooper, L. and Drabble, R. (1982) 'Police perception of crime', *British Journal of Criminology* 22: 1.

Boesel, D. and Rossi, P. (1971) *Cities Under Siege, Anatomy of the Ghetto Riots 1964–1968*, New York: Basic Books.

Bogolmony, R. (1976) 'Street patrol: the decision to stop a citizen', *Criminal Law Bulletin* 12: 5.

Bottoms, A., Mawby, R. and Walker, M. (1987) 'A localized crime survey in contrasting areas of a city', *British Journal of Criminology* 27(2): 125.

Bowden, M. (1982) *Community Watch, Bridgend*, Bridgend: South Wales Constabulary.

Bowden, T. (1978) *Beyond the Limits of the Law*, Harmondsworth: Penguin.

Box, S. (1981) *Deviancy Reality and Society*, London: Holt, Rinehart and Winston.

Boydstun, J. (1975) *San Diego Field Interrogation Study: Final Report*, Washington DC: Police Foundation.

Bridges, L. (1981) 'Keeping the lid on: British urban social policy 1975–81', *Race and Class* 23(2) and (3): Autumn.

Bridges, L. and Bunyan, T. (1983) 'Britain's new urban policing strategy: the Police and Criminal Evidence Bill in context', *Journal of Law and Society* 10: 85.

Bright, J. (1987) 'Community safety, crime prevention and the local authority' in P. Wilmott (ed.), *Policing and the Community*, London: Policy Studies Institute.

Bright, J. and Husain, S. (1990) 'Conclusion', in S. Husain and J. Bright (eds), *Neighbourhood Watch and the Police*, Swindon: Crime Concern.

Broderick, J. (1973) *Police in a Time of Change*, Morristown, NJ: General Learning.

Brogden, A. (1981) 'Sus is dead: what about "Sas"', *New Community* 9: 44.

Brodgen, M. (1982) *The Police: Autonomy and Consent*, London and New York: Academic Press.

—— (1985) 'Stopping the people: crime control versus social control', in J. Baxter and L. Koffman (eds), *Police: The Constitution and the Community*, Abingdon: Professional Books.

Brogden, M., Jefferson, T. and Walklate, S. (1988) *Introducing Policework*, London: Unwin Hyman.

Brown, D. and Iles, S. (1985) *Community Constables: A Study of a Policing Initiative*, Home Office Research and Planning Unit Paper No. 30, London: Home Office.

Brown, J. (1979) 'Community policing', *Police Review* 6 July: 1050.

Brown, M. (1981) *Working the Street*, New York: Russell Sage.

Bulmer, M. (1986) *Neighbours*, Cambridge: Cambridge University Press.

Butler, A. (1982) *An Examination of the Influence of Training and Work*

*Experience on the Attitudes and Perceptions of Police Officers*, mimeo, Bramshill: Police Staff College.

Cain, M. (1973) *Society and the Policeman's Role*, London: Routledge and Kegan Paul.

—— (1979) 'Trends in the sociology of police work' *International Journal of Sociology of Law* 7(2): 143.

Campbell, D. (1980) 'Society under surveillance', in P. Hain (ed.), *Policing the Police*, vol. 2, London: Calder.

—— (1990) 'The forces of prejudice', *Guardian* (Society), 31 October.

Centre for Contemporary Cultural Studies (1982) *The Empire Strikes Back*, London: Hutchinson.

Chambers, G. and Millar, A. (1983) *Investigating Sexual Assault*, Edinburgh: Scottish Office.

Chatterton, M. (1976) 'Police in social control', in J. King (ed.), *Control Without Custody*, Cropwood Papers No. 7, Cambridge: Institute of Criminology.

—— (1983) 'Police work and assault charges', in M. Punch (ed.), *Control in the Police Organization*, Cambridge, Mass.: MIT Press.

Chevigny, P. (1969) *Police Power*, New York: Pantheon.

Clark, J. (1965) 'Isolation of the police: a comparison of the British and American situations', *Journal of Criminal Law, Criminology and Police Science* 56: 3.

Clarke, M. (1990) *Business Crime: Its Nature and Control*, Cambridge: Polity Press.

Clarke, R. and Mayhew, P. (1980) *Designing Out Crime*, London: Home Office.

Clinard, M. (1978) *Cities With Little Crime*, Cambridge: Cambridge University Press.

Cochrane, R. and Butler, A. (1980) 'The values of police officers, recruits and civilians in England', *Journal of Police Science and Administration* 1980: 8.

Cohen, P. (1979) 'Policing the working-class city', in B. Fine, R. Kinsey, J. Lea, S. Picciotto and J. Young (eds), *Capitalism and the Rule of Law*, London: Hutchinson.

Cohen, S. (1979) 'The punitive city: notes on the dispersal of social control', *Contemporary Crises* 3: 339.

Coleman, A. (1985) *Utopia on Trial*, London: Hilary Shipman.

Colman, A. and Gorman, L. (1982) 'Conservatism, dogmatism and authoritarianism in British police officers', *Sociology* 16(1): 1.

Conklin, J. (1975) *The Impact of Crime*, New York: Macmillan.

Costa, J. (1984) *Abuse of the Elderly*, Cambridge, Mass.: Lexington Books.

Crawford, A., Jones, T., Woodhouse, T. and Young, J. (1990) *Second Islington Crime Survey*, Middlesex Polytechnic: Centre for Criminology.

Cray, E. (1972) *The Enemy in the Streets*, New York: Anchor.

Cumming, E., Cumming, I. and Edell, L. (1965) 'The policeman as guide, philosopher and friend', *Social Problems* 12: 3.

Cunningham, J. (1990) 'Thieving in the city', *Guardian*, 20 December.

Davis, J. (1989) 'From "rookeries" to "communities": race, poverty and policing in London, 1850–1985', *History Workshop* 27: 66.

Ditton, J. and Duffy, J. (1983) 'Bias in the newspaper reporting of crime news', *British Journal of Criminology* 23: 159.

Dixon, D., Bottomley, A., Coleman, C., Gill, M. and Wall, D. (1989) 'Reality and rules in the construction and regulation of police suspicion', *International Journal of the Sociology of Law* 17: 185.

Dobash, R. and Dobash, R. (1979) *Violence Against Wives*, London: Open Books.

Donajgrodski, A. (ed.) (1977) *Social Control in Nineteenth Century Britain*, London: Croom Helm.

Donnison, H., Scola, J. and Thomas, P. (1986) *Neighbourhood Watch: Policing the People*, London: Libertarian Research and Education Trust.

Doob, A. and MacDonald, G. (1979) 'Television viewing and the fear of victimization', *Journal of Personality and Social Psychology* 37: 170.

Du Bow, F. and Emmons, D. (1981) 'The community hypothesis' in D. Lewis (ed.), *Reactions to Crime*, Beverly Hills, Calif.: Sage.

Dunhill, C. (ed.) (1989) *The Boys in Blue*, London: Virago.

Durkheim, E. (1933) *The Divisions of Labor in Society*, translated and edited by G. Simpson, New York: Macmillan.

East, R. (1987) 'Police brutality: lessons of the Holloway Road assault', *New Law Journal* 137: 1010.

Ekblom, P. and Heal, K. (1982) *The Police Response to Calls from the Public*, Research and Planning Unit Paper No. 9, London: Home Office.

Ericson, R. (1982) *Reproducing Order: A Study of Police Patrol Work*, Toronto: Toronto University Press.

Farley, R., Schuman, H., Bianchi, S., Colasanto, D. and Hatchett, S. (1978) 'Chocolate City, Vanilla Suburbs', *Social Science Research* 7: 319.

Field, S. (1990) *Trends in Crime and Their Interpretation*, Home Office Research Study No. 119, London: HMSO.

Field, S. and Southgate, P. (1982) *Public Disorder*, London: Home Office Research Unit.

Fielding, N. (1988a) 'Competence and Culture in the Police', *Sociology* 22(1): 45.

—— (1988b) *Joining Forces: Police Training, Socialization, and Occupational Competence*, London: Routledge.

Fielding, N., Kemp, C. and Norris, C. (1989) 'Constraints on the practice of community policing', in R. Morgan and D. Smith (eds), *Coming to Terms with Policing: Perspectives on Policy*, London: Routledge.

Fink, J. and Sealy, L. (1974) *The Community and the Police*, New York: Wiley.

Fisher, C. and Mawby, R. (1982) 'Juvenile delinquency and police discretion in an inner-city area', *British Journal of Criminology* 22: 63.

Foster, J. (1989) 'Two stations: an ethnographic study of policing in the inner city' in D. Downes (ed.), *Crime and the City*, London: Macmillan.

Foucault, M. (1979) *Discipline and Punish*, New York: Vintage Books.

Frankenberg, R. (1966) *Communities in Britain*, Harmondsworth: Penguin.

Furstenberg, F. (1972) 'Fear of crime and its effects on citizen behavior', in A. Biderman (ed.), *Crime and Justice: a symposium*, New York: Nailburg.

Garofalo, J. (1977) *Public Opinion About Crime: the Attitudes of Victims and*

*Nonvictims in Selected Cities*, Washington DC: US Government Printing Office.

—— (1981) 'The fear of crime: causes and consequences', *Journal of Criminal Law and Criminology* 72: 839.

Garofalo, J. and McLeod, M. (1988) *Improving the Use and Effectiveness of Neighborhood Watch Programs: Research in Action*, Washington DC: National Institute of Justice.

—— (1989) 'The structure and operation of neighborhood watch programs in the United States', *Crime and Delinquency* 35: 326.

Gilroy, P. and Sim, J. (1987) 'Law, order, and the state of the Left', in P. Scraton (ed.), *Law, Order and the Authoritarian State*, Milton Keynes: Open University Press.

Goldsmith, J. and Tomas, N. (1974) 'Crimes against the elderly: a continuing national crisis', *Ageing* 236: 10.

Gordon, M. and Heath, L. (1981) 'The news business, crime and fear', in D. Lewis (ed.), *Reactions to Crime*, Beverly Hills, Calif.: Sage.

Gordon, P. (1983) *White Law*, London: Pluto Press.

—— (1984) 'Community policing: towards the local police state?', *Critical Social Policy* 10: 39.

—— (1987) 'Community policing: towards the local police state', in P. Scraton (ed.), *Law, Order and the Authoritarian State*, Milton Keynes: Open University Press.

Grade, M. (1989) *Report of the Working Group on the Fear of Crime* (The Grade Report), Home Office Standing Conference on Crime Prevention, London: HMSO.

Graef, R. (1989) *Talking Blues*, London: Collins Harvill.

Gramsci, A. (1986) *Selections From the Prison Notebooks of Antonio Gramsci*, edited and translated by Q. Hoare and G. N. Smith, London: Lawrence and Wishart.

Greater London Council (1984) *Racial Harassment in London*, London: Greater London Council.

Greenberg, S, Rohe, W. and Williams, J. (1985) *Informal Citizen Action and Crime Prevention at the Neighbourhood Level: Synthesis and Assessment of the Research*, Washington DC: US Department of Justice, National Institute of Justice.

Grimshaw, R. and Jefferson, T. (1987) *Interpreting Policework: Policy and Practice in Forms of Beat Policing*, London: Allen and Unwin.

Hall, R. (1985) *Ask Any Woman*, Bristol: Falling Wall Press.

Hall, S. (1979) *Drifting into a Law and Order Society*, London: Cobden Trust.

Hall, S., Critcher, C., Jefferson, T., Clarke, J. and Roberts, B. (1978) *Policing the Crisis*, London: Macmillan.

Hanmer, J. and Saunders, S. (1984) *Well-Founded Fear*, London: Hutchinson.

Harris, M. (1983) 'The media muggings', *New Society*, 31 March.

Heal, K., Tarling, R. and Burrows, J. (eds) (1985) *Policing Today*, London: HMSO.

Heidensohn, F. (1989) *Crime and Society*, London: Macmillan.

Henig, J. (1984) *Citizens Against Crime: an Assessment of the Neighborhood*

*Watch Program in Washington, D.C.*, Washington, DC: George Washington University, Center for Washington Area Studies.

Hibberd, M. (1985) *The Colville Crime Survey*, London: Police Foundation.

Hilliard, B. (1987) 'Holloway Road – some unfinished business', *New Law Journal* 137: 1035.

Holdaway, S. (ed.) (1979) *The British Police*, London: Edward Arnold.

—— (1983) *Inside the British Police*, Oxford: Basil Blackwell.

Home Office (1967a) *Circular Number 142/1967. Equipment for New Systems of Policing*, London: HMSO.

—— (1967b) *Report of the Working Party on Operational Efficiency and Management*, London: HMSO.

—— (1989) *The Response to Racial Attacks and Harassment*, London: HMSO.

Horton, C. (1989) 'Good practice and evaluating policing', in R. Morgan and D. Smith (eds), *Coming to Terms with Policing: Perspectives on Policy*, London: Routledge.

Hough, M. and Mayhew, P. (1983) *The British Crime Survey: First Report*, Home Office Research Study No. 76, London: HMSO.

—— (1985) *Taking Account of Crime: Key Findings from the Second British Crime Survey*, Home Office Research Study No. 85, London: HMSO.

Hunte, J. (1966) *Nigger Hunting in England*, London: West Indian Standing Conference.

Husain, S. (1988) *Neighbourhood Watch in England and Wales: a Locational Analysis*, Crime Prevention Unit Paper No. 12, London: HMSO.

—— (1990) 'Resources for scheme support', in S. Husain and J. Bright (eds), *Neighbourhood Watch and the Police*, Swindon: Crime Concern.

Husain, S. and Bright, J. (eds) (1990) *Neighbourhood Watch and the Police*, Swindon: Crime Concern.

Iadocola, P. (1985) 'Community crime control strategies', *Crime and Social Justice* 25: 140.

Ignatieff, M. (1983) 'Law and order in a city of strangers', *New Statesman*, 27 May.

Institute of Race Relations (1979) *Police Against Black People*, London: Institute of Race Relations.

—— (1987) *Policing Against Black People*, London: Institute of Race Relations.

Institute for Social Research (1975) *Public Safety: Quality of Life in Detroit Metropolitan Area*, Ann Arbor: University of Michigan, Survey Research Center.

Jaycock, V. (1978) 'The elderly's fear of crime: rational or irrational', *Victimology* 3: 329.

Jefferson, T. (1990) *The Case Against Paramilitary Policing*, Milton Keynes: Open University Press.

Jennings, A. and Lashmar, P. (1990) 'The wall of silence that refuses to fall', *Guardian*, 13 August.

Jones, J. (1980) *Organisational Aspects of Police Behaviour*, Farnborough: Gower.

Jones, S. (1986) *Policewomen and Equality*, London: Macmillan.

Jones, T., McClean, B. and Young, J. (1986) *The Islington Crime Survey*, Aldershot: Gower.

Kelling, G. (1986) 'Neighbourhood crime control and the police: a view of the American experience', in K. Heal and G. Laycock (eds) *Situational Crime Prevention: from Theory into Practice*, London: HMSO.

Kelling, G., Pate, T., Dieckman, D. and Brown, C. (1974) *The Kansas City Preventive Patrol Experiment: a Technical Report*, Washington DC: The Police Foundation.

Kelly, L. (1987) 'The continuum of sexual violence', in J. Hanmer and M. Maynard (eds), *Women, Violence and Social Control*, London: Macmillan.

Kettle, M. (1983) 'Fallible facts', *The Sunday Times*, 27 March.

Kettle, M. and Hodges, L. (1982) *Uprising*, London: Pan Books.

King, M. (1989) 'Social crime prevention à la Thatcher', *The Howard Journal* 28(4): 291.

Kinsey, R. (1984) *Merseyside Crime Survey: First Report*, Liverpool: Merseyside County Council.

—— (1985) *Merseyside Crime and Police Surveys: Final Report*, Liverpool: Merseyside County Council.

Kinsey, R., Lea, J. and Young, J. (1986) *Losing the Fight Against Crime*, Oxford: Basil Blackwell.

Kobrin, S. and Schuerman, L. (1981) *Interaction Between Neighborhood Change and Criminal Activity*, Los Angeles: University of Southern California, Social Science Research Institute.

Lambert, J. (1970) *Crime, Police and Race Relations*, Oxford: Oxford University Press.

Landau, S. (1981) 'Juveniles and the police', *British Journal of Criminology* 21: 1.

Landau, S. and Nathan, G. (1983) 'Selecting delinquents for cautioning in the London Metropolitan area', *British Journal of Criminology* 23: 2.

Law, I. and Henfry, J. (1981) *A History of Race and Racism in Liverpool 1660–1950*, Liverpool: Liverpool Community Relations Council.

Lea, J. (1986) 'Policing racism: some theories and their policy implications' in R. Mathews and J. Young (eds), *Confronting Crime*, London: Sage.

Lea, J. and Young, J. (1984) *What is to be Done About Law and Order?*, Harmondsworth: Penguin.

Lee, J. (1981) 'Some structural aspects of police deviance in relations with minority groups', in C. Shearing (ed.), *Organisational Police Deviance: its Structure and Control*, Toronto: Butterworths.

Lundman, R. (ed.) (1980) *Police Behavior*, New York: Oxford University Press.

Lundman, R., Sykes, R. and Clark, J. (1978) 'Police control of juveniles', *Journal of Research in Crime and Delinquency* 15: 212.

McBarnet, D. (1981) *Conviction*, London: Macmillan.

McConville, M. (1983) 'Search of persons and premises: new data from London', *Criminal Law Review* 1983: 605.

McConville, M., Sanders, A. and Leng, R. (1991) *The Case for the Prosecution*, London: Routledge.

McIntyre, J. (1967) 'Public attitudes towards crime and law enforcement', *Annals of the American Academy of Political and Social Science* 374: 34.

McNamara, J. (1967) 'Uncertainties in police work' in D. Bordua (ed.), *The Police*, New York: Wiley.

McPherson, M. and Silloway, G. (1987) 'The implementation process: effort and response' in A. Pate, M. McPherson and G. Silloway (eds), *The Minneapolis Community Crime Prevention Experiment*, Draft Evaluation Report, Washington, DC: Police Foundation.

Maguire, M. (1982) *Burglary in a Dwelling*, London: Heinemann.

Maguire, M. and Corbett, C. (1987) *The Effects of Crime and the Work of Victim Support Schemes*, Aldershot: Gower.

Malik, K. (1986) 'Crime, police and people: a reply to Trevor Jones and Jock Young', *New Society*, 14 February: 294.

Manning, P. (1977) *Police Work*, Cambridge, Mass.: MIT Press.

—— (1979) 'The social control of police work', in S. Holdaway (ed.), *The British Police*, London: Edward Arnold.

Manwaring-White, S. (1983) *The Policing Revolution: Police Technology, Democracy and Liberty in Britain*, Brighton: Harvester Press.

Martin, J. and Wilson, G. (1967) *The Police: a Study in Manpower*, London: Heinemann.

Marx, G. (1987) 'Yes sir, that's my daddy: when children turn in parents', *Student Lawyer* 15: 8.

—— (1989) 'Commentary: some trends and issues in citizen involvement in the law enforcement process', *Crime and Delinquency* 35(3): 500.

Mathieson, T. (1980) 'The future of control systems: the case of Norway', *International Journal of the Sociology of Law* 8: 149.

Mawby, R. and Gill, M. (1987) *Crime Victims: Needs, Services and the Voluntary Sector*, London: Tavistock.

Maxfield, M. (1984) *Fear of Crime in England and Wales*, Home Office Research Study No. 78, London: HMSO.

Mayhew, P., Elliott, D. and Dowds, L. (1989) *The 1988 British Crime Survey*, London: HMSO.

Miller, W. (1977) *Cops and Bobbies*, Chicago: Chicago University Press.

Minogue, T. (1990) 'Putting real crime on prime time', *Guardian*, 3 September.

More, W. (1976) *The American Police*, St Paul, Minn.: West Publishing.

MORI (1989) *British Public Opinion*, London: Market and Opinion Research International.

Moss, D. and Bucknall, R. (1982) *1982 Public Attitude Survey: Report*, Northampton: Northamptonshire Police Management Services.

Muir, J. (1977) *Police: Streetcorner Politicians*, Chicago: Chicago University Press.

Newby, H. (1979) *England's Green and Pleasant Land*, London: Allen Lane.

Newman, O. (1972) *Defensible Space: People and Design in the Violent City*, London: Architectural Press.

Norrie, A. and Adelman, S. (1988) '"Consensual authoritarianism" and criminal justice in Thatcher's Britain', *Journal of Law and Society* 16(1): 112.

Northamptonshire Police (1985) *Community Watch: Evaluation Report*, Northampton: Northampton Police.

Nuttall, C. (1988) 'Crime Prevention in Canada', in T. Hope and M. Shaw (eds), *Communities and Crime Reduction*, London: HMSO.

O'Leary, J. and Wood, G. (1984) *A Review of the Experimental 'Neighbourhood watch Scheme' Holmcroft/Tillington*, Stafford: Staffordshire Constabulary.

Pearce, F. (1973) 'Crime, corporations and the American social order', in I. Taylor and L. Taylor (eds), *Politics and Deviance*, Harmondsworth: Penguin.

Pearson, G. (1983a) *Hooligan: a History of Respectable Fears*, London: Macmillan.

―― (1983b) 'The Barclay Report and community social work: Samuel Smiles revisited?', *Critical Social Policy* 2(3): 78.

―― (1989) 'A Jekyll in the classroom, a Hyde in the street: Queen Victoria's hooligans', in D. Downes (ed.), *Crime and the City*, London: Macmillan.

Pearson, G., Sampson, A., Blagg, H., Stubbs, P. and Smith, D. (1989) 'Policing racism', in R. Morgan and D. Smith (eds), *Coming to Terms with Policing*, London: Routledge.

Peirce, G. (1982) 'Unleashing an uncritical press', *Guardian*, 15 March.

Police Foundation (1981) *The Newark Foot Patrol Experiment*, Washington DC: Police Foundation.

Policy Studies Institute (1983) *Police and People in London* 4, London: PSI.

Poulantzas, N. (1969) 'The problem of the capitalist state', *New Left Review* 58: 67.

Power, A. (1981) 'How to rescue council housing', *New Society*, 4 June.

―― (1988) *Property Before People*, London: Allen and Unwin.

Punch, M. (1979) *Policing the Inner City*, London: Macmillan.

―― (1983) *Control in the Police Organisation*, Cambridge, Mass.: MIT Press.

Punch, M. and Naylor, T. (1973) 'The police: a social service', *New Society* 24: 358.

Rees, A. (1950) *Life in the Welsh Countryside*, Cardiff: University of Wales Press.

Reiman, J. (1979) *The Rich Get Rich and the Poor Get Poorer*, New York: Wiley.

Reiner, R. (1978) *The Blue-Coated Worker*, Cambridge: Cambridge University Press.

―― (1985) *The Politics of the Police*, Brighton: Wheatsheaf Books.

Reiss, A. (1971) *The Police and the Public*, New Haven: Yale University Press.

Renvoize, J. (1982) *Incest: a Family Pattern*, London: Routledge and Kegan Paul.

Reppetto, T. (1974) *Residential Crime*, Cambridge, Mass.: Ballinger.

Riger, S., Gordon, M. and Lebailly, R. (1978) 'Women's fear of crime: from blaming to restraining the victim', *Victimology: an International Journal* 3: 274.

Rollo, J. (1980) 'The special patrol group' in P. Hain, M. Kettle, D. Campbell and J. Rollo (eds), *Policing the Police*, vol. 2, London: John Calder.

Rose, D. (1991) 'Ten years on and another city is on the brink of riot', *The Observer*, 7 April.

Rosenbaum, D. (1988) 'A critical eye on neighbourhood watch: does it reduce crime and fear?', in T. Hope and M. Shaw (eds), *Communities and Crime Reduction*, London: HMSO.

Rosenbaum, D., Lewis, D. and Grant, J. (1986) 'Neighborhood-based crime prevention: assessing the efficacy of community organizing in Chicago', in D. Rosenbaum (ed.), *Community Crime Prevention: Does It Work?*, Beverly Hills, Calif.: Sage.

Rossi, P., Berk, R. and Eidson, B. (1974) *The Roots of Urban Discontent*, New York: Wiley.

Rossi, P., Waite, E., Rose, C. and Berk, R. (1974) 'The seriousness of crimes: normative structure and individual differences', *American Sociological Review* 39: 224.

Royal Commission on the Police (1962) *Final Report*, Cmnd. 1728, London: HMSO.

Rubinstein, J. (1973) *City Police*, New York: Ballantine.

Rumbaut, R. and Bittner, E. (1979) 'Changing conceptions of the police role: a sociological review', in N. Morris and M. Tonry (eds), *Crime and Justice: an Annual Review*, vol. 1, Chicago: Chicago University Press.

Russell, D. (1982) *Rape in Marriage*, New York: Macmillan.

—— (1984) *Sexual Exploitation*, Beverly Hills, Calif.: Sage.

St Johnson, E. (1978) *One Policeman's Story*, Chichester: Barry Rose.

Sampson A., Stubbs, P., Smith, D., Pearson, G. and Blagg, H. (1988) 'Crime, localities and the multi-agency approach', *British Journal of Criminology* 28: 478.

Scarman, Lord (1981) *The Scarman Report: the Brixton Disorders 10–12 April 1981*, Harmondsworth: Penguin.

Scheingold, S. (1990) 'The politicization of street crime', in S. Silbey and A. Sarat (eds), *Studies in Law, Politics and Society: a Research Annual*, London: Jai Press.

Schneider, A. (1986) 'Neighborhood-based anti-burglary strategies: an analysis of public and private benefits from the Portland program', in D. Rosenbaum (ed.), *Community Crime Prevention: Does it Work?*, Beverly Hills, Calif.: Sage.

Scraton, P. (1982) 'Institutionalized racism in the Merseyside Police', in D. Cowell (ed.), *Policing the Riots*, London: Junction Books.

—— (1985) *The State of the Police*, London: Pluto Press.

Shapland, J. (1982) *The Victim in the Criminal Justice System*, Home Office Research Bulletin No. 14, London: Home Office Research and Planning Unit.

Shapland, J. and Vagg, J. (1987) 'Policing by the public and policing by the police', in P. Willmott (ed.), *Policing and the Community*, London: Policy Studies Institute.

Shapland, J., Willmore, J. and Duff, P. (1985) *Victims in the Criminal Justice System*, Aldershot: Gower.

Shaw, M. and Williamson, W. (1972) 'Public attitudes to the police', *The Criminologist* 7: 26.

Shearing, C. (1981a) 'Subterranean processes in the maintenance of power', *Canadian Review of Sociology and Anthropology* 18: 3.

—— (1981b) 'Deviance and conformity in the reproduction of order', in

C. Shearing (ed.), *Organizational Police Deviance: its Structure and Control*, Toronto: Butterworths.

Silver, A. (1967) 'The demand for order in civil society', in D. Bordua (ed.), *The Police*, New York: Wiley.

Silverman, R. and Kennedy, L. (1984) 'Loneliness, satisfaction and fear of crime', *Canadian Journal of Criminology* 27: 1.

Sim, J. (1990) *Medical Power in Prisons*, Milton Keynes: Open University Press.

Sim, J., Scraton, P. and Gordon, P. (1987) 'Introduction: crime, the state and critical analysis', in P. Scraton (ed.), *Law, Order and the Authoritarian State*, Milton Keynes: Open University Press.

Skogan, W. (1977) 'Public policy and fear of crime in large American cities', in J. Gardiner (ed.) *Public Law and Public Policy*, New York: Praeger.

—— (1981) 'On attitudes and behaviors', in D. Lewis (ed.), *Reactions to Crime*, Beverly Hills, Calif.: Sage.

—— (1984) 'Reporting crimes to the police: the status of world research', *Journal of Research in Crime and Delinquency* 21: 113.

—— (1986) 'Fear of crime and neighborhood change', in A. Reiss and M. Tonry (eds), *Crime and Justice: a Review of Research*, vol. 8, Chicago: University of Chicago Press.

—— (1987) 'Community organizations and crime', in M. Tonry and N. Morris (eds), *Crime and Justice: a Review of Research*, vol. 10, Chicago: University of Chicago Press.

—— (1989) 'Communities, crime and neighborhood organization', *Crime and Delinquency* 35(3): 437.

—— (1990) *The Police and the Public in England and Wales: a British Crime Survey Report*, Home Office Research Study No. 117, London: HMSO.

Skogan, W. and Maxfield, M. (1981) *Coping With Crime*, Beverly Hills, Calif.: Sage.

Skolnick, J. (1966) *Justice Without Trial*, New York: Wiley.

Skolnick, J. and Bayley, D. (1986) *The New Blue Line: Police Innovation in Six American Cities*, New York: Free Press.

Smith, D. (1987) 'The police and the idea of community', in P. Willmott (ed.), *Policing and the Community*, London: Policy Studies Institute.

Smith, D. and Visher, C. (1981) 'Street level justice: situational determinants of police arrest decisions', *Social Problems* 29(2): 167.

Smith, L. (1984) *Neighbourhood Watch: a Note on Implementation*, London: Home Office Crime Prevention Unit.

Smithers, A., Hills, S. and Silvester, G. (1990) *Graduates in the Police Service*, Manchester: Manchester University, School of Education.

Solomos, J. (1988) *Black Youth, Racism and the State*, Cambridge: Cambridge University Press.

—— (1989) *Race and Racism in Contemporary Britain*, London: Macmillan.

Southgate, P. (1982) *Police Probationer Training in Race Relations*, London: Home Office Research Unit.

Southgate, P. and Ekblom, P. (1984) *Contacts Between Police and Public*, London: Home Office Research Unit.

—— (1986) *Police–Public Encounters*, Home Office Research Study No. 90, London: HMSO.

Sparks, R., Genn, H. and Dodd, D. (1977) *Surveying Victims*, London: Wiley.

Stanko, E. (1984) *Intimate Intrusions*, London: Routledge and Kegan Paul.

—— (1988) 'Fear of crime and the myth of the safe home', in M. Borad and K. Yüo (eds), *Feminist Perspectives on Wife Abuse*, London: Sage.

Steedman, C. (1984) *Policing the Victorian Community*, London: Routledge.

Stevens, P. and Willis, C. (1979) *Race Crime and Arrests*, London: Home Office Research Unit.

Stoddard, E. (1968) 'The informal "code" of police deviance: a group approach to "blue-coat crime"', *Journal of Criminal Law, Criminology and Police Science* 59(2): 201.

Storch, R. (1975) 'The plague of Blue Locusts: police reform and popular resistance in Northern England 1840–57', *International Review of Social History* 20: 61.

Sykes, R. and Clark, J. (1975) 'A theory of deference exchange in police-civilian encounters', *American Journal of Sociology* 81: 584.

Sykes, R., Fox, J. and Clark, J. (1976) 'A socio-legal theory of police discretion' in A. Niederhoffer and A. Blumberg (eds), *The Ambivalent Force*, Hinsdale, Ill.: Dryden Press.

Taub, R., Taylor, D., Dunham, J. (1981) 'Neighborhoods and safety' in D. Lewis (ed.), *Reactions to Crime*, Beverly Hills, Calif.: Sage.

—— (1984) *Paths of Neighborhoods Change*, Chicago: University of Chicago Press.

Taylor, P. (1983) 'How Hendon cadets are wooed away from racialism', *Police*, 1983: 22.

Tchaikovsky, C. (1989) 'The inappropriate women', in C. Dunhill (ed.), *The Boys in Blue*, London: Virago.

Trotman, M., Russell, J., George, D. and Jenner, R. (1984) *Review of Neighbourhood Watch on No. 1 Area*, London: Metropolitan Police.

Tuck, M. and Southgate, P. (1981) *Ethnic Minorities, Crime and Policing*, Home Office Research Study No. 70, London: HMSO.

Turner, B. and Barker, P. (1983) *Study Tour of the United States of America: 7th March 1983 to 21st March 1983*, (2 vols), London: Metropolitan Police.

Tyler, T. (1980) 'Impact of directly and indirectly experienced events: the origin of crime-related judgements and behaviors', *Journal of Personality and Social Psychology*, 39: 13.

—— (1984) 'Assessing the risk of crime victimization: the integration of personal victimization experience and socially transmitted information', *Journal of Social Issues* 40(1): 27.

van Maanen, J. (1974) 'Working the street: a developmental view of police behavior', in H. Jacob (ed.), *The Potential for Reform of Criminal Justice*, Beverly Hills, Calif.: Sage.

—— (1977) 'Experiencing organization: notes on the meaning of careers and socialization', in J. van Maanen (ed.), *Organizational Careers: Some New Perspectives*, New York: Wiley.

Veater, P. (1984) *Evaluation of Kingsdown Neighbourhood Watch Project, Bristol*, Bristol: Avon and Somerset Constabulary.

Vincent, C. (1979) *Policeman*, Toronto: Gage.

Walker, M. (1978) 'Measuring the seriousness of crime', *British Journal of Criminology* 18(4): 348.

Walker, N. (1987) *Crime and Criminology*, Oxford: Oxford University Press.

Walklate, S. (1989) *Victimology: The Victim and the Criminal Justice Process*, London: Unwin Hyman.

Walsh, D. (1980) *Break-ins: Burglary from Private Houses*, London: Constable.

Waltham Forest Council (1990) *Beneath the Surface: an Inquiry into Racial Harassment in the London Borough of Waltham Forest*, Waltham Forest: Waltham Forest Council.

Ward, T. (1984) 'Armchair policing: a review of *What is to Be Done About Law and Order*', *The Abolitionist* 17(2): 35.

—— (1986) *Death and Disorder*, London: Inquest.

Washnis, G. (1976) *Citizen Involvement in Crime Prevention*, London: Lexington Books.

Weatheritt, M. (1983) 'Community policing: does it work and how do we know?', in T. Bennett (ed.), *The Future of Policing*, Cropwood Conference Series No. 15, Cambridge: University of Cambridge.

—— (1986) *Innovations in Policing*, London: Croom Helm.

—— (1987) 'Community policing now', in P. Willmott (ed.), *Policing and the Community*, London: Policy Studies Institute.

Westley, W. (1970) *Violence and the Police*, Cambridge, Mass.: MIT Press.

West Midlands Police (1982) *Resource Experiments, Volume 1: Main Report, Volume II: Statistical Tables*, West Midlands Police, Management Services Department, mimeo.

Whitaker, C. (1986) *Crime Prevention Measures*, Bureau of Justice Statistics Special Report, Washington, DC: US Department of Justice.

Williams, W. (1956) *The Sociology of an English Village: Gosforth*, London: Routledge.

Willis, C. (1983) *The Use, Effectiveness and Impact of Police Stop and Search Powers*, Research and Planning Unit Paper No. 15, London: Home Office.

Wilson, J. (1968) *Varieties of Police Behavior*, Cambridge, Mass. : Harvard University Press.

—— (1975) *Thinking About Crime*, New York: Basic Books.

Wilson, J. and Kelling, G. (1982) 'Broken windows', *Atlantic Monthly* 249: 29.

Winchester, S. and Jackson, H. (1982) *Residential Burlgary: the Limits of Prevention*, Home Office Research Study No. 82, London: HMSO.

Yin, P. (1980) 'Fear of crime among the elderly', *Social Problems* 27: 492.

Young, J. (1971) 'The role of the police as amplifiers of deviancy', in S. Cohen (ed.), *Images of Deviance*, Harmondsworth: Penguin.

Young, M. (1991) *An Inside Job*, Oxford: Clarendon Press.

# Name index

Adelman, S. 233
Alderson, J. 32, 116, 141
Aldridge, R. 227
Alex, N. 159
Anderton, K. 3, 221
Audit Commission 225

Bains, S. 93
Balbus, I. 233
Baldwin, R. 32
Banton, M. 31, 148, 235
Barker, P. 3
Bayley, D. 3, 33, 166, 187, 208
Bennett, T. 17, 94, 95, 105, 106, 170, 221, 247
Bent, A. 187
Benyon, J. 48, 210
Bittner, E. 16, 148, 233, 235
Black D. 170, 171, 181
Blom-Cooper, L. 75
Boesel, D. 231
Bogolmony, R. 170
Bottoms, A. 66
Bowden, M. 3
Bowden, T. 233
Box, S. 70, 75
Boydstun, J. 170
Bridges, L. 11, 235
Bright, J. 6, 9, 144, 225
British Crime Surveys 18, 19, 20, 21, 24, 28, 43, 57, 58, 68, 90, 93, 96–7
Broderick, J. 222
Brogden, A. 170
Brogden, M. 17, 47, 58, 109, 172,

212, 228, 236, 240, 241
Brown, D. 119
Brown, J. 141
Brown, M. 222
Bucknall, R. 32
Bulmer, M. 85, 223
Bunyan, T. 11, 235
Butler, A. 187
Byford, L. 4

Cain, M. 147, 148, 150, 153, 156, 166, 213
Campbell, D. 11, 169
Centre for Contemporary Cultural Studies 243
Chambers, G. 52
Chatterton, M. 148
Chevigny, P. 203
Clark, J. 159, 170
Clarke, M. 70
Clarke, R. 93
Clinard, M. 228
Cochrane, R. 187
Cohen, P. 202, 235, 241
Cohen, S. 85, 142
Coleman, A. 225
Colman, A. 187
Conklin, J. 80, 114
Corbett, C. 55, 56
Costa, J. 54
Crawford, A. 17, 46, 51, 59, 82, 95, 106, 107
Cray, E. 189
Cumming, E. 235
Cunningham, J. 227

# Subject index